How Drinking Can Be Good for You

How Drinking Can Be Good for You

(originally published as *Why Drinking Can Be Good for You*)

MORRIS CHAFETZ, M.D.

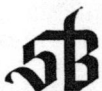

A SCARBOROUGH BOOK
STEIN AND DAY/*Publishers*/New York

FIRST SCARBOROUGH BOOKS EDITION 1978
How Drinking Can Be Good for You was originally
published in hardcover as *Why Drinking Can Be Good for You*
by Stein and Day/*Publishers*.

Portions of the text were originally
published by the *Johns Hopkins Magazine*, © 1976,
under the title "Carry Nation Had a Drinking Problem."
Copyright © 1976 by Morris E. Chafetz
Library of Congress Catalog Card No. 76-15934
All rights reserved
Designed by David Miller
Printed in the United States of America
Stein and Day/*Publishers*/Scarborough House,
Briarcliff Manor, N.Y. 10510
ISBN 0-8128-2477-6

DEDICATION

To M (of M & M)
I am sad to know that
The flower cannot see its beauty
The sunset cannot realize its glory
The infant cannot sense its future
The steel cannot feel its strength
or the furnace know its warmth
but I exalt that moment when
exquisite beauty graced my eyes
roaring glory touched my presence
unlimited future soared my horizon
limitless strength steeled my character
lifewarmth filled my soul
what more is there to say!

ACKNOWLEDGMENTS

Modesty is not one of my virtues unless I sit down to write a book. The organization and discipline a book requires just don't fit well with my personality. I am therefore in greater debt to many people than most authors.

I need to publicly thank Elise Hancock, able editor of the *Johns Hopkins Magazine*, whose persistence overwhelmed my reluctance to do the article "Carry Nation Had a Drinking Problem," which was the genesis of this book. My son Gary, an able author in his own right, interrupted his own writing to help organize his dad's. The organization of the book is, in the main, his idea. My son Marc and his friend Andrea Barkan gave generously of their ideas and suggestions.

Joyce Bartoo, of the National Clearinghouse for Alcohol Information, and Terry Bellicha, the director of the Clearinghouse, responded beyond the call of duty to my requests for material. My colleague Diana MacArthur furnished tidbits of insight that were helpful. The drinking diaries were devised in collaboration with my colleague Tom Harford. Joy Hall, my secretary, did yeowoman service in deciphering unbelievably illegible handwriting to type the manuscript, as did Sally Boyd and Dolores West.

My wife Marion's suggestions were sprightly and encouraging. I cannot claim, as do many other authors, that she struggled over the manuscript with me. She did not, and for good reason. How can a woman feel fresh enough to be critical about the writings of a man with whom she has shared the ups and downs of life for over thirty years? Her sensibility in always preventing me from taking myself too seriously in speaking to a serious subject is more valuable than I can express.

To my publisher, Stein and Day, and my editor, Eve Tulipan, my gratitude for recognizing that it was about time our society moved toward comfort and guilt-free experiences with drinking.

Morris E. Chafetz
Washington, D.C.

Contents

Carry Nation Had a Drinking Problem	11
The Best of Drinking	15
Persistent Notions	21
The Facts	31
Physical Effects	39
The Hangover	47
Alcohol and Your Health	51
Alcohol and Your Feelings	59
Alcohol and Other Drugs	63
You and Alcohol and Other People	67
Your Drinking Heritage	73
On the Job	81
Your Children	87
Drinking and Driving	95
The Law	99
Alcoholism	103
Diagnosis	111
Treatment	115
Prevention	125
Personal Drinking Records	129
Steps and Actions	153
Appendixes	165
Index	187

CARRY NATION HAD A DRINKING PROBLEM

Winston Churchill, when reproached by his wife about his love of liquor, once responded, "Clemmie, I have taken more good from alcohol than alcohol has taken from me." It's a salutary reminder—especially now, when almost any action we take seems fraught with risk and peril. Our water's undrinkable, our air is unbreatheable, our food causes cancer, or so we're told. We have enough to worry about.

I have devoted most of my professional life to the problems of alcohol and its abuse, most recently as director of the National Institute on Alcohol Abuse and Alcoholism. So I've spent much of my time trumpeting the fact—which most of us would rather not know—that alcohol is in fact a drug, and that alcohol problems, by any measure, are the most serious drug-abuse problems this nation faces. But still I must contend, with Sir Winston, that alcohol has done more good than harm. For when it is used safely it helps us answer our very human need to be in communication with others, the need to sometimes break out a bit, let go, and soar. And there is a safe way to drink.

We don't often talk about it, though. It seems we Americans always delight in focusing on the negative side of things. It seems strange to me as a psychiatrist that my colleagues and I can define pathology very easily, but the only way we can describe normalcy is, lamely, as the absence of pathology. This is particularly true in the field of alcohol abuse and alcoholism. We can talk about people who have serious problems with alcohol, but we're less prepared to speak to the issue of the majority of people who drink and, by and large, derive only the benefits of alcohol. Books, learned papers, popular articles by the score have defined, described, and offered solutions for the problems of alcohol abuse. Reformers thunder against the evils of drink. And those who enjoy even moderate drinking feel they can't admit to it without a wink and a wicked grin. Almost no one can say, simply, "Sometimes drinking can be good for you."

Why don't we talk about the benefits to be found in alcohol? I think it's partly because many of us are not very well informed on the subject. Then we don't go after the facts because we hesitate to ask questions about drinking. That might seem like admitting to a "problem" with alcohol. The difficulty is that we always approach a discussion of the *use* of alcohol as if it automatically meant *abuse*. Problem drinking is not the same as social drinking, and I believe that when we learn to make that crucial distinction we will have fewer problems connected with alcohol.

Taking that clear-eyed view will not be easy. Study after study has shown that people in the United States are very uncomfortable about drinking. We're so ambivalent and guilt-ridden about it that one can only conclude that we feel there's something deeply wrong with taking alcohol. Indeed, our many jokes on the subject are telltale, for jokes are a usually "safe" way to ventilate deeper worries or to give social sanction to something about which we feel concerned or guilty. Why is this country so uptight about drinking?

We find it very upsetting to see someone out of control; this threatens our own sense of control. And when we see an alcoholic, we really want to get rid of that unpleasant sight. It makes us fearful that we could become alcoholics, too. When we feel threatened, we retaliate. We become moralistic, judgmental, vindictive toward drinkers, preoccupied with drinking.

And how preoccupied we are. We spend a good deal of time

talking about drinking, thinking about it, worrying about it, looking forward to it. Look at the advertisements for alcohol. The message usually seems to be that you work your tail off all day long so that you can get to that beer or that drink. Alcohol is portrayed not as a small pleasure but as one of life's great rewards.

This preoccupation itself can be called a problem with drinking. I don't think you have to drink to be an alcoholic. I think Carry Nation was an alcoholic—a nondrinking alcoholic. She couldn't take care of her daughter, couldn't live with her husband because she was so obsessed with the Demon Rum. Didn't she have an alcohol problem?

On the other hand, Winston Churchill, by all reports, did drink an enormous amount, but some of us would like to drink as much if we could accomplish as much as he did. Sir Winston seems to have used alcohol in a way that amused and pleased him. Apparently it did not interfere with his functioning. He did not appear disquieted by his drinking—although his wife admonished him a bit—and he did live a long and fruitful life.

So it seems that problems with alcohol have as much to do with attitude as with amount consumed. Still, there is a scientifically defined safe amount we can drink, and most people do best when they stay within it.

There are, indeed, risks in taking alcohol, and my years of study in the field have made me acutely aware of them. But anything that affects human beings has a potential for harm. In excess, even oxygen and water, those essentials of life, can kill. Life itself is a risk, and I suspect the only sure way to be completely safe is to be dead.

With each passing birthday I become surer and surer of less and less. I am sure only that I don't want to admonish, to advise, to control, or to tell another human being how to live. I want merely to share some of the things I know with those who care to hear them. I want to dispel the myths and discuss the physical, psychological, and cultural facts as I understand them both about safe drinking and about problem drinking.

You must make your own decision about the risk taking. You may decide not to drink at all. But if you choose to drink and you have made the decision armed with facts and free of guilt, you can, like Winston Churchill, take more good than harm from alcohol.

The Best of Drinking

Getting the most from alcohol—the pleasure without the pain—is easy. It depends on knowing why you react to a drink as you do. A number of things contribute to your response. First in importance, of course, is the chemical action of the alcohol in your body and your physical condition. But the place, the time, the companions, your mood and expectations—all play a vital part in making alcohol work well for you.

How alcohol works in the body

Most people don't realize that alcohol is an anesthetic, not a stimulant. In moderate amounts it appears to stimulate because it inhibits the "new" part of the brain—the part that records new learning, judgment, and social controls—as well as the brain centers that make us aware of exhaustion and discomfort. A little alcohol makes us feel physically able and emotionally freer. With increasing doses, however, alcohol puts these brain centers to sleep. Then the "older" part of the brain—the center for our more primitive, less socialized impulses—begins to take over. Sufficient dosage can put us to sleep for keeps, by anesthetizing the centers that control breathing and heartbeat.

Alcohol is a quick-acting drug. About 20 percent is absorbed through the stomach, goes immediately into the bloodstream, and travels to the brain. The remainder is absorbed through the intestine.

How much to drink

Most people can enjoy the benefits of alcohol and avoid the pain if they drink no more than one and a half ounces of absolute alcohol per day. That would be three 1-ounce drinks of 100-proof whiskey (it should be drunk diluted), or four 8-ounce glasses of beer or half a bottle of table wine. Researchers from all over the world have independently defined this amount as safe.

The figure, based on recent research, is not really new. In 1862 Sir Francis Anstie, a British psychiatrist, made public Anstie's Law of Safe Drinking, which *also* stated that one and a half ounces of absolute alcohol per day was the upper limit of moderate drinking. (Sir Francis, a man ahead of his time, was responsible, in 1870, for establishing the first women's medical school in Great Britain, and served as that school's first dean.)

Anstie's limit is an upper limit, and a statistical average that cannot be applied to all individuals. For some people, even one drop of alcohol is a drop too much. Quantities may also vary depending on body weight, physical and psychological condition.

Neither Anstie's Law nor our findings permit saving up one day's ration so you can drink more the next day.

How to drink

The way you drink is extremely important. You should always sip slowly. Alcohol is a highly unusual foodstuff in that 20 percent of it is absorbed directly from the stomach into the bloodstream without having to go through any digestive processes. Gulping alcohol produces a sudden, marked rise in the alcohol level in the blood and hence in the brain. Even if subsequent drinks are taken slowly, you will tend to have an unusually strong reaction to the dose.

Besides sipping slowly, how can you keep your system from overreacting to alcohol? You can dilute the alcohol with plenty of ice to further slow the rush into the bloodstream. Food in your stomach, preferably protein or fatty foods, taken before you drink is most effective in slowing alcohol's invasion of the bloodstream and brain. An experienced drinker knows that, all things being equal, the same dose of alcohol taken with food in the stomach will provide a different, more pleasant outcome than alcohol on an empty stomach.

When to drink

Alcohol does the most for you when you choose the time, place, and circumstances of drinking rather carefully. Now, obviously, if you are going to be writing, driving, filling out a tax form, or engaged in any other highly complex mental or physical activity, it scarcely seems appropriate to be under the influence of an anesthetic drug. On the other hand, if you're going to be sharing a meal or enjoying human interchange, just sitting around in a relaxed way, then alcohol can be a terrific adjunct to the essential human experience of socializing. It's then that alcohol is at its best, a true servant of man.

The Chinese sip their alcohol, savoring each drop as a gift of God, and they drink to celebrate their mutual interdependence. Drunkenness and alcoholism are almost unknown in China. Having observed safe and healthy drinking practices in many parts of the world, I've learned that where alcohol is used in the Chinese style, people generally reap its great gifts while avoiding its pain.

Where to drink

It's best to drink in a relaxed setting—in your own home, at a restaurant with friends, on any comfortable occasion for socializing. Now, standing up while drinking is not a relaxing way to drink, and certainly drinking alone is not a relaxing way to drink. Indeed, if I had to come up with an unhealthy drinking situation, it would be the American cocktail party. It is a contribution to the world's drinking practices that I wish we had not made.

Standing around uncomfortably in a crush of people, most of whom we don't know, makes us want to gulp that first drink. People like to think that the alcohol at cocktail parties makes it easier to get acquainted, and cite the fact that strangers will frequently pour out intimate details of their lives at these parties. In my judgment these outpourings are proof of just the opposite. A relative stranger sharing intimacies so freely in such an inopportune circumstance is, in a sense, speaking to himself because his inhibitions have been put to sleep. He is not relating to you.

Pick the right drinking companions

Good drinking depends on good company. It's really best not to take alcohol when you're physically or emotionally upset, lonely, or in need of solace. Alcohol is no substitute for another person. It is true that alcohol's neat anesthetic effect will dull the pain of loneliness. It will free us to dream a little, to transcend the routine of reality. But what better safety measure for our flight into worlds splashed with color and enthusiasm than sharing that beauty and insight with at least one other human being?

In other words, do not drink alone.

Just as important, look twice at the people you choose to drink with, for they will play a part in the effect the drink has on you. Regardless of where and how you drink, what you expect from alcohol is what you get, and the expectations and tolerances of the people around you will help determine your own response—irrespective of dose. In other words, if you're part of a group that wants to act drunk, even with small doses you'll feel drunk.

It's best to drink with people who set expectations that are socially useful and not destructive. Americans fail in this regard.

When we Americans drink, we celebrate independence and individuality. The image we worship is a frontier person who can stand alone against threatening natural forces, depending on no one, controlling his or her own destiny. Unfortunately, we try to express this ideal of ruggedness through our drinking. As a corollary, when Americans drink, there is a focus on prowess, on "how much one can hold"; too many Americans drink to prove something about themselves.

In a nutshell

Responsible drinking is taking alcohol as just a part of, rather than the reason for, an activity. To focus on drinking as an end in and of itself is the wrong way to go about it.

Responsible drinking includes making sure there is food in our stomachs before we drink. It means we sip our drinks slowly in a relaxed, comfortable setting, usually in the company of other people. We neither seek nor welcome drunkenness. We do not drink more than Anstie's limit.

We pay attention to how we respond to the alcohol if we are tense, tired, or emotionally upset. We're not uncomfortable around people who choose not to drink. We're not uncomfortable if there are times when we choose not to drink.

I guess the cocktail of responsible drinking contains the following ingredients: a jigger of self-respect combined with a dash of common sense poured over cubes of knowledge and stirred well with people.

Persistent Notions

In America the subject of drinking and alcohol has long invited intense interest, often colored with a good deal of emotionalism. As a result, questionable facts based on shaky information have passed into our folklore as truths. Some, indeed, are true, but many should be consigned to the world of myth, and forgotten. Here are a few of each kind.

Alcohol is an aphrodisiac

Alcohol is an indirect aphrodisiac. It does not directly affect sites or hormones that stimulate us (if they, in fact, exist). But in moderate doses it anesthetizes our control centers and allows natural sexual inclinations to surface. It lets us hear those gods of hope and beauty and tenderness imprisoned in all of us. We are willing—even daring. Certainly, then, alcohol has aphrodisiac gifts.

But all gifts have a price. With more than moderate amounts of alcohol, desire persists but performance dies. We shouldn't be surprised. Sex demands sensitivity, and heavy anesthesia deadens the senses. Heavy drinkers have lousy sex lives.

There is one slightly positive link between heavy drinking and sex. Men troubled by premature ejaculations—hair-trigger orgasms—find that heavy doses of alcohol slow down the reaction. The catch is that they may be too drunk to appreciate what's happening. Substituting an alcoholic illness for a treatable embarrassment is the wrong therapy for the condition.

Alcoholism is hereditary

Most studies confirm that alcoholism is learned and not inherited. Those studies that seem to point to a genetic cause are flawed because the definition of alcoholism is flawed. There is no fixed set of symptoms that I know of that can be identified as a disease that passes down through the generations.

But alcoholism does run in families. Study after study has shown that in alcohol clinics 70 percent of the patients had significant people in their lives with alcohol problems. We know that children of alcoholic parents are at greater than average risk of developing alcoholism if the right kinds of circumstances prevail. That does not mean they're sure to develop alcoholism. Caution, not fear, is indicated.

If our parents were alcoholic, the betting odds on potential alcoholism are higher on us than on the child of the normal drinker. Risks and odds are generalities—they have no specific or individual significances. Here's an example: When we flip a coin, the odds are 50-50 that it will come up heads. But if we've flipped it ten times, and ten times it's come up tails, the odds are still no better than 50-50 that the eleventh flip will be heads. The previous flips have no relevance to the next flip.

All evidence shows that children of alcoholic parents are at greater general risk. But there is no specific, individual danger. As a matter of fact, with caution and sensible, moderate use, they may be better off than others because they have been alerted to the hazards.

There are two dangers in the heredity theory. First, it reinforces the widespread and unjustified sense of futility about trying to treat alcoholic people. Second, by insisting on a hereditary factor, we introduce that strong barrier of hope and change, the self-fulfilling prophecy.

Be convinced that something will happen, and chances are it will. If a child is raised to believe that his genes propel him toward alcoholism, he has a strong head start. Who among us believes we have any chance to change our destiny when heredity is involved?

Learned family behavior, however, leaves us alternatives. What is learned can be unlearned.

Societies, when frustrated by a problem, seduce scientists into finding a genetic quirk to explain what seemingly can't be changed. Alcoholism, in my opinion and experience, is not inevitable. It can be treated and prevented.

Few women become alcoholics

I wish I could say that, but it would not be true. Women, like men, have always had trouble with alcohol. And their problem is increasing.

Many people believe that an alcoholic woman is sicker and

more difficult to treat than an alcoholic man. This belief is based on the false notion that there is something different in women alcoholics that makes them sicker. The problem here is not in women, but in us men. We're so sure that alcoholism is the outcome of too much manliness with booze that we can't hear the women in our midst screaming for help. Because we need to hold onto things masculine—even a disease like alcoholism—women have to become very sick indeed before we can bear to notice that they have alcohol problems.

We all know that the acknowledged rights and roles of women are changing. But without their own measure of success, women striking out into new fields aim for accepted male marks of achievement. Heavy drinking, unhappily, is one. Alcohol, once the medicine for the lonely, bored housewife is becoming the rite of passage for women seeking success in the "man's world."

There is no cure for alcoholism

If we doctors had to deliver cures to earn our income, we'd all be on welfare! The truth is that we cure very little; we don't cure diabetes, heart disease, colds, ulcers, cancer, high blood pressure, or hundreds of other afflictions. If our patients are lucky, we make them hurt less and function better than they did before they came to see us.

Alcoholism, like other common conditions, can't be cured, but it is very treatable. A study completed in 1975 showed a better than 70 percent recovery rate in the populations of government-supported clinics. Study after study reaffirms how treatable—easily treatable—alcoholic people are. The only untreatable part of alcoholism is you and me. Our fixed ideas and expectations concerning alcoholic people load the dice against them. Such expectations applied to other conditions would first stigmatize the afflicted and then make them feel helpless and hopeless.

We are all prisoners of our own experience. Whatever we have learned through observing a few alcoholic people, we apply to all alcoholic people. My experience is twofold: (1) I've never met an alcoholic who, given an alternative, would choose to be an alcoholic. (2) I've never met an alcoholic person who, given the treatment that was right for him or her, could not hurt less and function better.

A recovered alcoholic should never drink again

In the best of all possible worlds, who can argue with that statement? And if you are a recovered alcoholic person and have a choice, I guess a guarantee that you'll never drink again means—in the classic sense—that you'll never have an alcoholic problem. That was the logic underlying Prohibition: Remove alcohol by law, and *poof!* no more alcohol problems in the nation. We know what that logic cost us.

I am not suggesting that alcoholic people try to drink. I've always told my patients, "After the misery you've gone through, why take the risk of finding out whether or not you can drink again? Alcohol is not a necessity of life."

That's sound advice, and many of us know of recovered alcoholics who have taken one drink and relapsed dramatically. Our individual experiences, however, do not negate the scientific studies that show that recovered alcoholics who abstain entirely during the recovery period are just as likely to relapse as those who take some alcohol during that period.

The greatest tragedy of the rigid rule against any alcohol ever for recovered alcoholics is that it scares off a great many people from early diagnosis and treatment. Often, when people notice something different about their drinking, they think, "I'm going to be *forever* set apart as a nondrinker in a drinking society." That drives them deeper into drink.

I have no rules of recovery for the patients I have served. They have to feel and function better according to *their* criteria. When I set criteria for recovery that are mine—not theirs—then the treatment is for me—not them.

Association with heavy drinkers will lead to a drinking problem

Chameleons take on the color of their surroundings; people are not much different. If you are surrounded by heavy drinkers, you do increase the risk of becoming one. (And most heavy drinkers, unless they change their drinking style, develop alcohol problems.) Those of us caught up with such associates can talk to them about our discomfort at the chemical barrier they raise between us. Let them know we want relationships with people, not substances.

If that approach fails, there is no need to continue to punish ourselves. Why risk developing a drinking problem for a non-relationship? If I continued in such a circumstance—and I had my rescue and omnipotence fantasies under control—I'd begin to wonder about myself. Maybe I'd find that I can relate to people only when they aren't really there.

Some businesses and professions require constant association with heavy drinkers. The trick here is to take one or two drinks with a mixer and follow it for the rest of the evening with mixer alone. At long drinking lunches the rule is: Dawdle. When neither technique works, remember there is a lot of self-respect and dignity in pleasantly refusing a drink.

A drink can kill a hangover

To kill a hangover with a drink is fighting fire with fire—things can get out of control. Now, there are two ways of getting hangovers: (1) Drink in a tense, uncomfortable situation, or when you yourself are tense and overwrought (you can experience a certain kind of tension even at parties where drinking is part of the fun). (2) Drink heavily, often. In each case a dose of alcohol may bring temporary morning-after relief.

In the first kind of hangover, a drink will block out the message of discomfort being sent to the brain and kill the misery. In the second, the victim is actually suffering early mild drug-withdrawal symptoms—tremor, sweating, sensitivity to light and sound, headache. A dose of the substance withdrawn will relieve the symptoms.

In both cases you pay for this relief later.

Alcoholics have addictive personalities

Studies have failed to support the thesis of an addictive personality. We are pretty good at pointing out certain features that already labeled addicts have in common. But when it comes to pointing out why others who also have these features cannot be clinically labeled addicted, we're not so successful. We certainly have not been able to use these common features to predict who will, and will not, develop an addiction syndrome.

The clinical definition of addiction is the development of withdrawal symptoms upon ceasing to take a substance. We are all addicted to something: work, or religion, or play. If we're honest with ourselves, we know that the prolonged withdrawal of some of our routines makes us uncomfortable.

When we are discomfited by the absence of our addictive mechanisms, we search for substitutes. Just as the person who is addicted to work goes on vacation and works hard at play, the alcoholic without alcohol will find a substitute. Both have addictions, but neither need be doomed to hopelessness by the label "addictive personality."

Coating the stomach with milk prevents drunkenness

It's not a bad practice. Milk will protect a stomach about to receive alcohol. The fat in milk slows absorption, and the fluid acts as a dilutant. Drinkers who are careful enough to take this precaution will most certainly be careful about drinking. Unless they think that once they've done it, they can throw all other cautions to the wind and drink fast and hard. Not so.

Alcohol kills brain cells and diminishes intelligence

Every second, in most parts of our bodies, millions of cells die; most to be replaced by new recruits. Brain cells die, too, and there is no methodologically sound study that conclusively shows that alcohol speeds up this natural process. If anything kills brain cells in abundance, it is more likely to be nonuse.

However, studies show that with moderate doses of alcohol, intelligence—as measured by the ability to solve complicated abstract problems—increases. In one experiment, highly intelligent, well-trained people solved problems in symbolic logic better with two drinks than without alcohol. At four drinks, they were at their normal level of performance; at six, much below.

Black coffee and a cold shower are the best ways to sober up

If I knew a quick way to sober us up, I'd be a rich man who had made an enormous social contribution. But there's no such thing as a free lunch. If you overdose with the drug alcohol, there is no way (save for a kidney dialysis machine) to clear your blood of alcohol except through the body's usual physiological and chemical processes (metabolism) that break down the foods we take in. Alcohol is destroyed at the rate of three-fourths of an ounce of absolute alcohol (about one average drink) per hour.

The caffeine in black coffee and the jolt of a cold shower may make us wide-awake drunks—but drunks we are. Alcohol's effects can be controlled only on the way in. After that, time is in command. We have one thing to decide: Are we safer as sleepy drunks or as wide-awake drunks?

Red wine will make you sicker than white wine

Too much of either will make us very sick. Although red wine is almost twice as acidic as white and contains more tannins, I do not believe a given amount of red wine will make you sicker than the same amount of white wine.

"Whiskey on beer, nothing to fear; beer on whiskey, mighty risky"

Taking beer first means that the first alcohol entering our bloodstream is diluted, and we know that's safer. Beer also has volume in the stomach, which slows the absorption of whiskey. So we'd have dilution and delay—all to the better.

The other way around, with the whiskey first—and I'm assuming the whiskey is taken straight (if the whiskey is well diluted, the ditty is meaningless)—means a concentrated rush of alcohol to the bloodstream that then gets reinforced and heightened by the alcohol in the beer. I guess that's why a straight shot of whiskey with a beer chaser is called a boilermaker—it's a drinking explosive.

Of course, consuming drinks in rapid succession—no matter which they are—is not a safe way to drink.

The Facts

Myths may be comfortable, but facts are more useful in coming to terms with drinking and alcohol. In this case what you know can definitely help you.

What is the pharmacologic action of alcohol?

Pharmacologically, alcohol is a central nervous system depressant drug. It is in the class of barbiturates, sedatives, and general anesthetic agents.

It has a dual effect. At very low doses the mild anesthesia of brain centers results indirectly in stimulation of functions. For example, the heartbeat increases, and there is increased energy. Alcohol's immediate and most important effect is upon the highest functions of the brain: thinking, learning, remembering, and making judgments. It is this slowing down of the tense, driven part of our brain that makes alcohol a delicious adjunct to socializing. But as the concentration of alcohol increases, depression of brain centers intensifies, resulting in sedation, narcosis, coma, and even death. Pharmacologic examples of the release, or excitement, stage are manifested by loss of social restraints, exhilaration, talkativeness, mood changes, and at times even emotional outbursts. At times the gait is unsteady, certain fine discriminations are lost, and speech is slightly slurred.

At high doses, reflex responses, visual acuity, and alertness are diminished. Visible drunkenness, with heavily slurred speech, confused thinking, and weaving gait, can be observed. At very high doses, most of us are anesthetized: difficult to arouse, incapable of voluntary action, and comatose.

Does body weight affect our reaction to alcohol?

Along with how much, how, what, and where we drink, we need to keep our body weight in mind. The person with more weight has more tissue in which alcohol is distributed. There is no hard-and-fast rule about how much more or less a given individual can take because so many factors enter into alcohol's effect upon us. The general rule of thumb: a man of 180 pounds can safely have three ounces of 86-proof liquor or sixteen ounces of beer in two hours. For each twenty pounds up or down from that median, you either add or subtract a half ounce. Therefore, the 240-pound man could consume four and a half ounces of spirits in two hours, whereas the 140-pound man should have only two ounces in two hours.

Women, due to their generally smaller bone structure and muscle mass, should take less than men.

Blood and brain, those tissues richest in water, get the highest concentration of alcohol. The lowest is found in muscle and fat.

Are alcohol calories the same as food calories?

Calories are units of heat energy given off by metabolic processes. The energy of alcohol calories is the same as that of other food calories, but alcohol's calories are different in other respects. First, they provide no minerals or chemicals essential for good nutrition. They are empty calories—quick, easy *zips*, but nothing more. Some beers and wines contain nutritious material, but I don't advocate them as a way of satisfying the nutritional needs of the body.

Second, alcohol calories can't be stored, so our bodies use them first. When alcohol has provided the energy we need before we take in food calories, we store the food calories and get fat. If we are trying to limit our calorie intake and depend only on alcohol as the source, we develop nutritional deficiency diseases, and they're not nice.

Is alcohol a hunger suppressant?

In moderate doses, alcohol livens the appetite for most people. Some doctors still prescribe it for patients who have lost their zest for eating.

Heavy doses of alcohol, on the other hand, tend to kill the desire to eat. First, when we need food, our body sends us hunger signals. If our ability to be aware of these signals is impaired by a heavy dose of anesthesia, we're unlikely to respond. Second, the calories of alcohol make us feel satisfied temporarily. And third, a stomach lining irritated by alcohol won't want to receive food.

How fast does alcohol take effect?

Alcohol is a fast-acting drug. A tiny bit gets into the blood by inhalation as you drink, but the first significant amount gets into the bloodstream from the stomach. Up to 20 percent may be absorbed this way. Minutes after the drink is swallowed, alcohol is well distributed throughout the body, since it requires no digestive action.

Is it better to dilute drinks?

With hard liquor, absolutely and always, unless, of course, it is a brandy or other drink that is to be sipped very slowly. The concentration of alcohol in our glass will be reflected in the concentration of alcohol in our bloodstream and brain. We should try to dilute well with plenty of ice and plain water. Wine and beer need not be diluted, of course, since they provide alcohol in a dilute form. Avoid carbonated mixers. They rush alcohol into the bloodstream because the gas creates pressure that forces the liquid quickly through the walls of the capillaries in the stomach lining. We're interested in comfortable drinking, not hard whacks.

Why does food "kill the kick"?

Food in the stomach slows the rate at which alcohol enters the intestine and bloodstream by mechanically covering the stomach wall, making capillaries (the quick way into the blood) less accessible. Food also slows absorption because it sponges up the alcohol and carries it, with the food, slowly through the digestive process. A slow rate of absorption allows the metabolic processes and brain to adapt. We don't overwhelm our systems.

Is alcohol habit-forming? Why aren't we all addicted?

If habit-forming means physiological addiction, then alcohol is habit-forming. We have to drink a lot over a long period of time to get physiologically addicted to alcohol. So most of us don't become addicted.

Contrary to common belief, taking addicting substances doesn't mean that we're almost immediately hooked. We have to work at getting addicted. Government reports tell us that there are people who use heroin intermittently and are *not* addicted. Heroin is a much more addicting drug than alcohol.

Do a twelve-ounce can of beer, an ounce of 100-proof rum, and six ounces of wine all contain the same amount of alcohol?

The form a drink comes in doesn't always tell you how much alcohol it contains. The twelve-ounce can of beer has the same alcoholic content as the ounce of 100-proof rum, the only difference between them is the volume in which we find them.

Six ounces of wine—if it is table wine—has 50 percent more alcohol than the twelve ounces of beer or the one ounce of rum. If it is six ounces of fortified wine (such as vermouth, sherry, or port), it contains about 75 percent more alcohol than the beer or rum.

In vodka we can find great variation—from 80-proof up to the Russian 150-proof. It's wise to know the alcoholic content of what we drink. We all should realize, too, that the alcoholic content of hard liquor is kept foolishly high because of federal laws. The standards of identity set by the government require that a product labeled gin, brandy, tequila, rum, vodka, scotch, or rye, and so on, must be at least 80-proof. Those less than 80-proof must have the word *diluted* printed on the label in conjunction with the statement of class (gin, vodka, and so on) in the same type size. This, needless to say, discourages manufacturers from marketing lower-proof products.

Is the alcohol stronger in certain drinks?

The alcohol in whiskey is not stronger than the same amount in wine. The differences in effect depend on the rate at which the alcohol reaches the brain. The person who drinks whiskey straight usually takes his quantity of alcohol in a period of minutes, while the wine or beer drinker, because of dilution and volume, will take a longer time to consume the same amount of alcohol. Even when the wine or beer drinker takes in more actual alcohol, the continuous oxidation and elimination of alcohol by the body over the longer time span makes for a lower blood alcohol concentration. Of course, well-diluted whiskey sipped slowly will have the same moderate effect as wine or beer.

What is denatured alcohol?

Denatured alcohol is ethyl alcohol—the alcohol we drink—which has been purposefully contaminated. Chemicals are added to ethyl alcohol to make it smell and taste awful. Denatured alcohol is used to make 128 commercial products from shellac to antifreeze. Industry contaminates the alcohol so that it will get used for its commercial purposes instead of for parties by the employees.

Is there a difference between rubbing alcohol and the alcohol we drink?

Rubbing alcohol is impotable alcohol. There are medical needs for alcohol solutions. Rubbing alcohol helps to bring down a fever, make the bedridden comfortable, and has many other external uses.

The form of alcohol used is isopropyl, not ethyl, alcohol. Isopropyl alcohol tastes terrible and will make you very sick if you drink it.

How do scientific studies compare the dangers of alcohol and marijuana use?

Most scientific studies would incriminate alcohol as being more dangerous with misuse than marijuana. Alcohol in large doses over a period of time is physiologically addicting. Marijuana is not. Heavy doses of alcohol increase the risk of developing certain cancers and neurological and muscle diseases. Marijuana does not. Alcohol in heavy doses is related to murders and other criminal activity. Marijuana generally is not. Alcohol in heavy doses is related to brain damage. Marijuana is not.

Aside from legal and emotional questions, we cannot escape the fact that, according to present knowledge, heavy alcohol misuse is much more serious than heavy marijuana use.

What does being "high" mean? What does alcohol do to make me feel and act this way?

Being "high" is when both feet are on the ground, yet we're flying because we've accumulated more alcohol in the body than can be metabolized in the steady state of three-fourths of an ounce of absolute alcohol per hour. When alcohol puts to sleep the higher brain centers affecting judgment, perception, and social controls, the deep brain centers take over. Perceptions dim, and we move from familiar patterns toward instinctual behavior. Landmarks are lost. It's like flying in an airplane without a horizon indicator. It's a giddy feeling. But we are discombobulated.

Physical Effects

Since alcohol is, in a sense, both a food and a drug, it can in both roles affect our weight, our sex life, and our appearance.

Why do I gain weight when I stop drinking?

If we stopped drinking and didn't substitute other things, we'd lose weight. But alcohol satisfies personal and social needs. That's the reason we've used it over the ages. And that's the reason we go on using it in spite of the problems it creates for a minority of drinkers.

Some people, whose love needs are not met, try to relieve their loneliness and pain with alcohol. Because alcohol anesthetizes the pain, they begin to feel that drinking gives them the comfort and satisfaction a close relationship with another person could offer. Some people drink because they have an unusual need for fluids (polydipsia). Still others need a great deal of oral stimulation. When alcohol is removed in any of these situations, substitutes are sought. No Alcoholics Anonymous meeting could hope to operate without barrels of coffee. Coffee—often with cream and sugar—and carbonated drinks by the gallon supply not only a lot of liquid but a lot of calories.

Along with the need for liquids, we also crave sweets when we stop drinking—especially chocolates. That's not going to help us hold the weight line, either.

My experience tells me, though, that the sensible moderate drinker who stops drinking will *not* usually gain weight.

Are some kinds of booze less fattening than others?

This is the kind of question that drives experts to overdrink. The frustration arises from calorie charts. I've never found two that use the same figures when they describe equivalent drinks. I suspect that the calorie determination depends on the taste of the determiners. If the beverage is to their liking, it's marked low. If they're not so wild about it, a high score is used.

We can assume that an average ounce of absolute alcohol provides us with 150 to 200 calories.

What about the "drinking man's diet"?

If you want to lose weight, I'd suggest that you give up drinking while dieting. Even small doses of alcohol put to sleep the control centers of recent memory and strict judgment. Those of us who, like Oscar Wilde, can resist anything but temptation had best not have our resolve weakened by alcohol when faced with food. It's hard enough to say a noble "No" when our determination is strong.

Alcohol is also an appetite stimulator. I can't imagine why any dieter would want to stimulate his or her appetite.

And the calories! Now, the "drinking man's diet" seems to promise we can continue to drink and still lose weight. That is also possible—witness the emaciated look of skid row alcoholic people.

Do drinkers have better sex lives than nondrinkers?

Drinking would be even more popular than it is today if this statement could be proved true. Certainly some alcohol advertising would like us to believe it, for Americans are inordinately preoccupied with achieving "better" sex. Better than what—the last one, the mythologized one, the advertised one, or the dreamed-about one? We still faithfully believe that a simple formula can solve complicated and sometimes difficult interpersonal relations and that "great" sex is the only mark of interpersonal success. I'm not knocking great sex; when all of the delicate sensitivities work, it's just that—great! But, like all the pleasures of life, it's temporary and can't be forced.

I believe moderate drinkers generally have better sex lives than nondrinkers. In sex I equate "better" with "freer." And except in people who can't stand the taste of alcohol or have bad physical reactions (headache, nausea), nondrinking is an expression of control. In taking alcohol we are implying that we are willing to give up a tiny bit of control. And since the right amount of freeing up means better sex, I think moderate drinkers have better sex lives than nondrinkers.

What causes a beer belly?

Beer is a high-calorie drink. The beer companies acknowledge this by promoting light beer, which is purported to contain fewer calories than regular beer. The heavy beer drinker gains a great deal of weight.

When we are young, our chests are tight and strong. Middle age begins when our chest shifts to our middle and starts to sag. Fat from any cause loves our middle. Presto: a beer belly. I suspect, too, that for those of us whose major recreational activity is sitting on a bar stool or before a television set guzzling beer, the lack of exercise hastens the collapse of the belly wall.

What causes a drinker's red nose?

One of the actions of alcohol is vasodilation. Vasodilation, or a widening of the openings of blood vessels, comes about because alcohol anesthetizes the centers in the brain that control the vessel walls, and permits them to relax.

Normally, when our surroundings are cold, our blood tends to pool up deep within our bodies to preserve heat. It's one of the reasons we turn blue—the blood has essentially fled from our skin surfaces. Vasodilation, on the other hand, causes the blood to reach surface areas in our bodies. (That is why we feel warm from a drink when we are cold; it is also the reason it is unwise to drink when we are to remain in frigid surroundings.)

The capillaries (the tiniest of blood vessels) are most exposed in the nose, and the nose is exposed to the elements.

Engorged, blood-rich capillaries exposed to cold or trauma often break, causing the red nose. This is not uncommon in frequent heavy drinkers, à la W. C. Fields. I suspect that Nature—in that way it has of mocking us—lights up red beacons on the noses of people who do not responsibly use and appreciate Nature's gift of alcohol.

Why do I get thirsty when I drink?

One of the popular myths is the full-bladder explanation: We lose a lot of water through the kidneys, and we are thirsty because of water loss. Another, that alcohol on the skin has an astringent action: Therefore, alcohol inside must dry us out, leaving unquenchable thirst.

The thirst of drinking is a product of shift—not loss or drying. Alcohol and its mineral content (especially sodium) causes the fluid within the cell structure to leave and flow into the intercellular spaces. When the cells contain less water, we feel thirsty. Taking fluids when we are thirsty is not so much for water replacement as it is to dilute the salts in the spaces between the cells so the electrolytic balance between space and cell again shifts and the fluid flows back into the cell.

Keep the alcohol well diluted and you won't feel thirsty.

When heavy drinkers stop drinking, why do they gorge themselves on sweets and drink enormous amounts of fluids?

The heavy drinker knows no bounds in his desire for fluids when he stops drinking. But this is not a passing phenomenon, similar to what we may experience after an evening of drinking. Quart after quart of liquid is consumed throughout the waking hours.

I can only guess at the reason. Since heavy drinking does cause water shifts in the body, prolonged heavy drinking produces prolonged shifts and local tissue addiction. The shift of fluids to the intercellular spaces is so constant that the expected rebound action does not take place. We need fluids perpetually. We did not notice this changed need when drinking heavily, because of the anesthetic effects of the alcohol.

The craving for sweets common to people who've given up drinking is not dissimilar. Eating sweets is a well-known substitute for love. Alcohol—in heavy doses—can make us think that we are feeling love and being loved even when it's far from true. Or it can dull the pain of feeling lonely and unloved. When alcohol is gone, sweets become the replacement for the comfort drinking formerly gave us.

Gorging on fluids and sweets provides another satisfaction. Some of us get a pleasurable sensation of fullness when our bladder or our stomach is bloated. There are psychiatric formulations that can explain it either as filling a need for love or as an expression of self-loathing.

It often happens that I have a couple of drinks and I don't get high. Why?

If all the steps of responsible drinking are followed, we shouldn't get high. We can feel good about the world, the people in it, and ourselves. Some people drink to get a high and achieve that delicate state between early intoxication and drunkenness. Not only is it difficult to get to, it is difficult to hold. Many drinkers who shoot for this goal go over the edge and get drunk.

A more logical question is: Why does a given dose of alcohol sometimes not provide the effect we've previously experienced with it? It might simply be a time when, terribly uptight and severely controlled, we've unconsciously set our will against letting anything affect us.

It may be the circumstances and the setting. All things being equal, the drinks with my best friend will produce one kind of effect in me, and the same number of drinks taken at a White House function would produce an entirely different effect. With my friend, I'll let go more, feel, and perhaps act, a little high. At the White House I'll remain in careful control.

These are times when what we expect and what we are allowed are important in determining alcohol's effect upon us.

Why do I get the "whirlies" when I lie down and close my eyes after drinking?

The merry-go-round effect with alcohol is hypotensive. We know that alcohol is a vasodilator. Although there is a very short period when the blood pressure rises after drinking (the heart control center's mild sleep after the initial drink causes a speedier heartbeat and consequently a slight rise in blood pressure), the vasodilation does cause it to fall a bit below its usual level. This lower blood pressure usually lasts as long as alcohol is affecting the brain.

Some people suffer what is known as postural hypotension. They don't need to be drinking. They can just be lying down. The phone rings, they jump to their feet with a start, and they've got the "whirlies." These people tend to the low side of blood pressure readings, and it's quite likely that even a little alcohol will make them dizzy. They don't even have to lie down.

But when you drink and lie down, the postural hypotension along with the vasodilation due to alcohol gives you the "whirlies."

Why do I get tipsy after three drinks, while my friend, who is short and skinny, needs ten to get tipsy?

Dose and size are one thing. Expectation and control are another.

You might be tipsy because you gulped three drinks in fifteen minutes on an empty stomach. Your short, skinny friend may take thirty to forty-five minutes with food in his stomach to finish each of his drinks. On the other hand, your friend may have a problem. He may need to keep tight control of himself so that neither he nor others will talk about the man who needs to down ten drinks.

And then there is the phenomenon of tolerance: increasing doses required to produce a previous effect. We don't fully understand it, but we see it.

We still have much to find out about the action of alcohol, but we do know one thing: Never envy a heavy drinker who does not seem to get tipsy. Alcoholism may be the next station on his train ride.

The Hangover

Try as we will to drink sensibly, there will probably come a day when we'll drink too much, or drink under the wrong conditions, and we'll be struck with that swift, just retribution—the hangover. What can we do about it?

What is a hangover?

Physiologically, hangover is due to fatigue. Heavy doses of alcohol so put our brain to sleep that we do not recognize and respond to the signals telling us that our nerves and muscles are exhausted. We push ourselves beyond our points of endurance because we have anesthetized the protecting warning systems in our brains. We've disrupted our bodily systems, and the nausea, gastritis, headache, and anxiety we experience are the rude awakening to what we could not be aware of when we were heavily overdosed.

Complications and specific discomforts are also related to the type of food eaten, the type of liquor drunk and its congener content (congeners are contaminants that add color, aroma, and flavor), and other physical and emotional influences—some understood, others not—that reinforce the miseries of hangover symptoms.

Why is a hangover?

A hangover is a misery worn like a badge. In spite of all the concoctions created to ease the suffering, in spite of the promise of untold riches for the person who conquers its blight, many Americans actually take pride in their hangovers—this proof of having had a "big night." Why else would we have them?

Watch some of us in the presence of a person in the vise of a hangover: the knowing smile; the kidding remark; and the complete acceptance of their debilitating state of misery.

I heard no easy familiarity with hangover in China, Israel, Spain, Italy, or Lebanon. Interestingly, the countries that focus on them are the countries with big or growing alcohol problems. It could be that other societies do have hangovers and just don't like to talk about them, but I doubt it.

In societies that place drink in the proper perspective and drink sensibly, there are few drinking problems and hangovers are rare. But where heavy is the name of the game, where getting drunk is O.K., where there's conflict, ambivalence, and guilt about drinking, hangovers become pandemic. And we're involved in "uptight" drinking. When we're tense and uptight while taking alcohol, we're more predisposed to hangover. When we're conflicted and guilty about alcohol, we're often ignorant about the drug and its effect, and foolish about how we use it.

Can hangovers be avoided?

Mild, occasional hangovers cannot be avoided. We can experience hangover symptoms (headaches, shakiness, and so on) without alcohol when we push ourselves too far—shutting out the signals that warn us: Enough. When we take a drink or two under these conditions, we will further close down the warning signals, push ourselves farther, and make our hangover discomfort worse. Alcohol seems to be the facilitator rather than the cause here.

How to treat a hangover

Since fatigue is the root cause of hangover, rest is the best therapy. There is no way to put off your body's need for plenty of rest to recover. If your stomach is not upset, aspirin will lessen the aches, pains, and headache common to hangover. Stay away from alcohol—it only delays the moment of reckoning. Abstinence for seventy-two hours with a mild hangover, and a week to ten days with severe hangover, is a very good idea.

Clear fluids are helpful. Some suggest whiffs of oxygen. All kinds of pills and concoctions are recommended, but to my knowledge no pill or chemical has been found that allows the body to do without rest once we've taken a lot of alcohol and pushed ourselves over the edge of our endurance.

How to avoid a hangover

If we think we are going to drink a lot, we should protect ourselves from the miseries of hangover. These few simple steps will help: Eat a decent amount of food before beginning to drink. Sip the first drink slowly for thirty to forty-five minutes. Sip well-diluted drinks while continuing to eat. Make sure you are in as relaxed a setting and emotional state as possible.

If we can put a man on the moon, why haven't we invented a pill to kill the hangover?

We *have* invented a "pill" to kill the hangover: perpetual, heavy doses of alcohol. But that may kill the sufferer, too.

I guess the awesomely sophisticated mechanical problems we solved to get to the moon are still less complex and easier to resolve than the problems surrounding the emotional responses of fear, loneliness, guilt, fantasies, the human state.

Hangover cures are unlikely to come until we cease being human and become mechanical.

Does switching drinks (for example, gin to bourbon to whiskey) or mixing them with carbonated liquids affect my hangover?

Switching drinks—in and of itself—does not cause hangovers. The culprits are the alcohol content and concentration, not the kind of drink. Some scientists contend that the congeners reinforce and intensify hangovers when they do begin.

Carbonation can contribute to the hangover. Carbonation speeds the alcohol into the bloodstream, and we know that speeding it in gives a high initial whack.

Alcohol and Your Health

Even one drink has measurable physical effects. In some conditions these effects provide a real medical benefit. Heavy drinking, of course, can cause chronic health problems or permanent damage.

If you drink moderately, will you live longer?

Statistically, according to the *Second Report on Alcohol & Health* done by the U.S. government in June 1974, moderate drinkers do live longer than ex-drinkers, heavy drinkers, and abstainers, apparently because moderate drinkers generally are the kind of people who enjoy social life and have life-enhancing interests. Statistically, moderate drinkers have less heart disease. Ex-drinkers have usually discontinued drinking because of complications arising from an illness. Heavy drinking causes many types of organic disturbance and disease, whereas moderate drinking does no harm to health, according to our present knowledge.

Most abstainers, according to some studies, don't drink for reasons of principle or because of health problems. Others abstain because they are "social dropouts"—they abstain from all the delights and challenges of life. Such general withdrawal may be related to dying younger and may partly explain the difference between the life spans of abstainers and moderate drinkers.

However, people are not generalizations, and hundreds of individual responses pop up to defy the statisticians. In one case the solace and support an abstainer finds in following his religious or ethical principles are more important to his well-being than a statistical probability that he will live longer if he drinks moderately. In the case of a severe alcoholic, even a drop of alcohol may trigger malignantly heavy drinking.

So the comforting statistic is there, but only you can decide whether it applies to you in your individual circumstances.

How does alcohol affect your heart?

Moderate drinkers seem to have less heart disease than heavy drinkers or abstainers. Moreover, persons with heart disease can benefit from moderate doses of alcohol. Many patients find that a little alcohol relieves the painful grip of angina pectoris and allows them to take fewer nitroglycerine tablets. Alcohol is a vasodilator—it opens the blood vessels, permitting the blood to flow more freely.

Its calming, analgesic qualities quiet the anxiety natural to the heart patient. It is not easy to live while wondering if every twinge of pain in the chest heralds disaster. Relaxation and sedation with mild doses of alcohol may speed the recovery of the cardiac patient.

Alcohol and the elderly

Disturbed digestion, aches and pains, feelings of isolation and uselessness, and the need for heavy doses of medication diminish in the elderly with occasional small doses of alcohol because of its mild anesthetic effect.

Is alcohol medication?

Alcohol serves as the basic ingredient in combination with other drugs in liquid medications and tonics. Historically, it was used alone in some cases. Before the age of antibiotics, physicians would prescribe small doses of whiskey for infants suffering from pneumonia. And, most certainly, if our movies or television can be believed, cowboy heroes could not have withstood the pain of a bullet extraction without heavy swigs of booze.

On chronic disease wards today it is used to ease the patients' discomfort and allows them to focus on something other than their illness.

Many a tonic advertised and sold as an over-the-counter medication to help your blood or relieve your infirmities owes its success in part to the alcohol in the mixture.

Does alcohol improve the appetite?

Alcohol can help stimulate the appetite because the brain's inhibitory centers are less alert. Sensations of fatigue, jaded taste, and nervous indigestion are silenced, and food begins to smell, look, and taste better. Certainly, alcohol weakens the will to resist eating.

Alcohol and digestion

Historically, small doses of alcohol have been taken before meals to aid digestion. Wine is particularly useful for this purpose.

The acid content of wine is close to the acidity of the gastric juices, so it is compatible with normal functioning. The mild anesthetic effect overcomes the "dry mouth" associated with stress or tension, and we salivate more freely. Salivation, in turn, reflexively triggers motility—the gentle motion that empties the stomach and is considered beneficial to digestion. One or two glasses of wine taken with a meal can produce this effect.

Heavy doses are another story, resulting in an irritated stomach wall, an increased concentration of alcohol, and an anesthetized stomach too sleepy to move or so overwrought it tightens up in a spasm.

Is it all right to drink a little when you have an ulcer?

You should not drink any alcohol if you have an ulcer. The raw, exposed stomach tissue does not take kindly to alcohol's action. It is foolish and dangerous to drink—even a little—when you have an ulcer.

Will alcohol help me sleep?

A small amount of alcohol taken about a half an hour before retiring can relieve tension and induce sleep. I do not recommend it as a daily practice because if you should need to increase the dose, the opposite outcome, poor sleep, may occur. After heavy doses of alcohol, you will sleep fitfully and wake up exhausted. This is due to a decrease of REM, or dreaming sleep. For reasons not yet fully understood, we need to dream a certain amount each night. When our REM sleep is blocked, our concentration and memory diminish and we feel anxious, tired, and irritable. Alcohol blocks REM sleep because it narcotizes (or anesthetizes) the control centers that regulate sleep and dreaming. Narcosis is not sleep.

Probably the best way to induce sleep is to forget about it. Read, work, watch TV, and don't fight for sleep. When we need sleep, we sleep. We all make a lot of fuss about getting enough sleep, but I've never heard of an insomniac dying for lack of it, and many people function perfectly with only a few hours a night.

How does drinking affect nutrition?

When we drink within Anstie's limits we affect our nutrition only a little. We may have a bit more fat floating around in our blood and even being deposited temporarily in our livers. Although the reason for the floating fat is not totally understood, it is considered to be due to the process of alcohol oxidation that releases an excess of hydrogen in the liver. The increase in hydrogen is thought to inhibit certain metabolic functions helpful in deriving energy from other sources, so the alcohol becomes the "preferred fuel" for energy. The hydrogen also frees fat from other parts of the body to float in the blood. This fat settles in the liver but disappears within twenty-four hours of the cessation of drinking. It is interesting to note that if the body doesn't use all the calories provided by alcohol, they do not get stored as fat, as do nutritional calories.

Heavy drinking is another matter. Floating fat is not all we have to worry about. We're so anesthetized that we don't eat; or, if we do, we don't eat properly or we vomit and lose food. We also upset the balance and the behavior of the metabolism and absorption of our gastric and intestinal system. We can't extract all the good nutrients that the consumed food has to offer. Heavy doses of alcohol are bad enough for us, but when heavy drinking causes nutritional deficiencies, the real complications of alcoholism set in.

Some contend that it is only the nutritional defects that lead to difficulty, and not the alcohol. I think this is a foolish differentiation. Even if we eat properly but drink heavily, we so upset complicated metabolic mechanisms that nutritional pandemonium breaks out.

Does a drinking spree present any special health hazards?

The steady, daily, moderate drinker is at lower risk of developing health problems with alcohol than the person who drinks sporadically but with a vengeance.

In my opinion, a spree of drunkenness constitutes a very real threat to your health.

What are the adverse physical effects of heavy drinking?

The brain, nerves, muscles, stomach, and throat can be affected. We do not know if the harm is done by nutritional deficiencies or by the heavy intake of alcohol directly. I believe that most investigators still buy nutritional interference rather than direct alcohol action. One thing we're all agreed on is that there is no known advantage to one's health afforded by *heavy* drinking.

Most investigators are not convinced that cirrhosis of the liver is caused directly by heavy doses of alcohol. In an interesting study by a New York group, thirteen baboons were fed large quantities of alcohol along with adequate diets. Two cirrhotic livers resulted. Unfortunately, the study could not measure whether or not the baboons' heavy alcoholic intake interfered with their ability to absorb the nutritious diet. The group claims its study proves direct effects because it controlled the experiment by a properly balanced diet. I'm not so sure. Whether or not these claims are correct, there is no doubt that heavy drinkers put their livers at risk, and all agree that if you drink heavily you are better off if you take an adequate nutritious diet.

Alcohol and Your Feelings

The goal of drinking—stated or otherwise—is to affect emotions. Through all of history, man has attempted to alter reality, to quiet fears and soothe anxieties through the use of chemical substances. Among the most commonly used has been alcohol. Since we cannot change this fact of the human condition, we're well advised to understand why alcohol affects us.

Why does alcohol make me feel more relaxed and uninhibited?

Tension and inhibitions are the work of the new part of the brain, the part most sensitive to alcohol.

When we take some alcohol, the activity of that brain center slows down. Social controls relax. We're less tense; we're less inhibited. We feel free. In a sense we might say we are a trifle less civilized and a trifle more ourselves. That's why most of us drink.

Why do I get *more* depressed if I drink?

I'd stop drinking if I got more depressed when I drank. Drinking is for reaching out, not for reaching in. The intensification of depression with drink means two things: The depression is serious, and the wiping away of surface control brings it out into the open. Help is needed.

Moreover, when alcohol increases depression, drinkers tend to take more and more alcohol as medication for the depression. There are many successful treatments for depression, so why make it worse with alcohol? Don't complicate a depression with a drinking problem.

During times of social turmoil and upheaval, is there an increase in the national consumption of alcohol?

Some studies confirm that during periods of national disturbances a nation, like a person, turns more to drink and alcohol consumption rates do rise.

Why do I occasionally feel that I *need* a drink?

Any of us who take alcohol will occasionally reach a point of exhaustion or tension that leads us to seek the anesthetic solace of alcohol. Occasionally feeling the need for a drink is an expression of the human experience.

If the world and its people were perfect, we would never feel we *needed* a drink. To need a drink is to put alcohol into a functional role that is potentially dangerous. If we frequently say "Boy, I *need* a drink," it's time to be cautious. It means we're moving toward a dependence on alcohol. If we need to be dependent, let's become dependent on something other than alcohol.

When we drink for the drug effect, we gradually require increasing doses to achieve the original response. That's how alcohol problems are made.

Why can I feel close to certain people I am fond of only when I've had something to drink?

Some of us have been raised in families where feelings and a show of warmth and closeness are not encouraged. These patterns of restrained response become so much a part of our being that even when we know intellectually that we want to feel close, we can't.

With moderate doses of alcohol and the release of social controls, the innate human impulse to be close to other people is not so frightening.

Alcohol and Other Drugs

Alcohol in combination with other drugs can have unexpected, often devastating, and sometimes lethal effects. We should never take alcohol with any medication or mood-altering drug without first finding out what those effects are likely to be.

Is mixing alcohol and drugs really that dangerous?

Many deaths are known to have been caused by the mixing of alcohol and other drugs. We suspect—but obviously don't know—that many unexplained deaths and accidents are also the result of mixing alcohol and other drugs.

Combining drugs can produce one of two outcomes. The first is called an additive response and is predictable; that is, half a dose of each drug in combination produces the equivalent effect of a full dose of each. The second, and more unpredictable, outcome is a synergistic or potentiating response: Combining two drugs that have a synergistic action produces two, three, or more times greater effect than a full dose of either or both together. Even small doses of alcohol (less than Anstie's limits) combined with other drugs (see page 169) can knock us temporarily or permanently on our tails. I recommend, strongly, that if you're taking any medication, you be extremely cautious in your drinking.

Which drugs are more dangerous with alcohol than others?

Physicians most commonly warn against using barbiturates, sedatives, and antihistamines in combination with alcohol, but the dangers of combining alcohol with any other medication can be serious. A detailed listing of drugs and their interaction with alcohol can be found in Appendix I. For quick reference see the chart in Appendix II.

Probably the best rule is to take no alcohol when you are on any medication; but since few of us exercise such stern self-discipline, it is well to know which are the most dangerous and the kind of reaction to each.

An interaction between alcohol and barbiturates or tranquilizers (not necessarily of a heavy dose) may cause or contribute to automobile or other kinds of accidents.

Other analgesic drugs, like the salicylates (such as aspirin or sodium salicylate) generally, with continuous use, tend to produce some bleeding in the stomach. And of course the irritation from alcohol may aggravate the condition. You can protect yourself by using buffered salicylate products and lining the stomach with food before taking them.

Heavy doses of alcohol in combination with salicylates can interrupt the blood-clotting mechanism in some people and cause hemorrhaging.

You and Alcohol and Other People

Alcohol can be a gentle catalyst for social interaction. It works best when you use it as a means of reaching out to others. Whether you use it poorly or well will depend on you, on the group you are with, on the job you hold, and possibly most of all on the society you live in.

The company you keep

We do not like to think about it, but most of us behave acceptably not because of rules, regulations, and laws, but because we want the affection and respect of a few individuals around us, and the limits of what they will or will not accept are quickly transmitted. We make sure, if we care to continue the relationships, that we do not go beyond these limits. Therefore, it is increasingly clear that if there is an individual in our group who misuses alcohol, in addition to asking what problem that person is dealing with, we need to ask what role the rest of us play in influencing him to try to solve his problems with alcohol.

Drinking together

Thousands of years ago, when people found the world even more mystifying than we do today, men and women lived in terror of the forces that seemed to control their fate. Alcohol not only mellowed the terror but made it possible to experience these forces comfortably and even to gain some sense of mastery over them. Thus, alcohol took its place in religious ritual.

Pagan religion, like modern religion, was partly social, a gathering for mutual support. Alcohol, too, became a part of the general culture. Soon it was used to ratify contracts, solemnize crownings, mark festive events, and confirm all rites of passage through life. Today we celebrate with alcohol the birth of a child, entry into college or a profession, hopes for a marriage or a new job, and new partnerships. Even death and the funeral's pain are softened by drinking.

Wine enhances a food's natural flavor, heightens its aroma, and increases one's gustatory pleasure. Alcohol's beneficence to the appetite is mentioned in the Bible. "Drink no longer water, but use a little wine for thy stomach's sake."

Expressions of hospitality, sociability, and conviviality would be incomplete in some circles without alcohol.

Alcohol in small doses allows the shy person to speak, the

sexually constricted to respond. Drinking can affirm affection and real friendship.

Group drinking often has a broader significance than the mere consumption of alcohol. Pubs in England are really social clubs for meeting and entertaining friends and acquaintances. Although skid row drinking groups usually meet as mutual sources of alcohol supply, they are also a mode of cohesiveness for these otherwise isolated people.

Whenever we drink chiefly to get in touch with other people, we are drinking for the best reason.

Why are people friendlier when they drink?

When we drink we are less self-conscious, less serious, less self-impressed. In moderate doses, alcohol becomes a leveler, a socializer. When alcohol gently nudges to sleep the stern forms of "new" brain control, the dormant humanistic impulses wake up. And we are friendlier.

Why is it that at some parties everyone has a good time, but no one gets drunk; while at other parties the *same* people get drunk and act like fools?

Each party is set up for its outcome. We transmit the message clearly. Serve no food, and we're saying alcohol is all. Top the drinks off just as soon as they dip below the rim, and we're saying alcohol is all. Push people to drink when they're not in the mood, and we're giving them the message: Drunk is in.

Serve food first, and then a drink or two. Don't delay dinner. Don't urge guests to drink. Make the seating arrangements conducive to conversation. Keep the noise level down. Keep the lights up. The focus is on people, not drink. Drink is the accompaniment, not the preoccupation. The message: How could we get drunk and act like fools in such a setting?

As we saw earlier, the basic influence at work here is

expectation. When we drink, we most often get the response we, or those around us, expect.

Why do I feel more comfortable at a party when others are making fools of themselves?

Some people are tragically self-conscious. They are, as one person put it, corseted in the belief that the lights and cameras are on them only. Yet they dread actual center-stage. If someone acts the fool at a party, they're more comfortable because the pressure is off them. They are not the focus; it has been shifted to the fool.

Why is it so hard to be at a cocktail party and not be drinking?

It's not unlike being at a movie and not looking. A party named after a drink implies a get-together just to drink. If you don't drink, you have to feel left out, especially if the host or other guests act as if you're being unsociable. It's difficult even for the strongest among us. The trick, of course, is to have *something* in a glass to sip on. I've included a list of drinks without alcohol on page 158 that will make it a bit easier.

Does peer pressure often make people drink?

We are all influenced by certain people whose respect, affection, and acceptance we desire and need. I don't call this peer pressure; I call it peer need.

All of us need the emotional and social support of other people. The people who are important to us set limits (formally or informally) as to how far we can go and what they'll tolerate. If the relationship is good, they do not force us to do things we don't really want to do. Instead, they share our views of the world, our cares, our pleasures. That sharing provides support, comfort, and a testing of reality. We all need this.

Pressure to drink or do anything else is neither caring nor sharing; it is using. Unfortunately, our peer needs sometimes make it very hard to resist destructive pressures.

What is the relationship between religion and drinking?

Religious affiliation often offers some protection against developing an alcohol problem. The dogma wholeheartedly accepted by members of a religious group is an interesting combination of personal conviction and peer pressure. In the denominations whose strictures against taking alcohol are especially strong, most of the young do not drink. But when they do, they are quite likely to develop alcohol problems.

Your Drinking Heritage

Each national or ethnic group, it seems, has its own general approach to drinking—the importance given to alcohol, the way it's used, the feelings toward drunkenness. The attitudes of the group shape the individual member's drinking patterns.

How is the American value system reflected in our drinking habits?

We are a country that revels in abundance. We produce and drive an enormous number of cars. Our food and resource production are enormous. We want television sets and telephones in every room. We consume prodigiously. And when we drink, some of us drink heavily.

What do the problem drinking nations have in common?

I don't know which of us (among the United States, France, Sweden, and the Soviet Union) is the Hertz, and which is the Avis. I do know that there are too many serious alcohol problems in all four countries. The United States, Sweden, and the Soviet Union suffer these problems for similar reasons—their people don't know how to drink. They drink fast and furiously; they use drinking to prove prowess; they focus on alcohol; they ascribe to it magical qualities that it doesn't deserve; they often drink without food; and drunkenness is implicitly and explicitly approved.

France's problem is somewhat different. French people, particularly the working class, honestly believe that water is unsafe and wine is good for the blood. They use wine to quench thirst as well as an accompaniment to meals and to sip for relaxation at interludes all day long. For many, the day routinely begins with cognac and coffee. Though the roaring drunk is rare, the quiet drunk is all too common, and alcohol problems are widespread.

How much does the average American drink?

We can know the per capita consumption of alcohol only through tax figures, and these figures can be misleading. Washington, D.C., for example, has the highest per capita consumption (it is twice the national rate, and this does not include the drinking in embassies, which is tax-free) in the United States. Do we have a capital of heavy drinkers? Not necessarily.

Washington has no rural area to dilute its population concentration. It is a convention and tourist center, and we tend to drink more, and more often, when at conventions or on vacation. Washington is a low-cost liquor spot, so bargain hunters come to the District from surrounding Virginia and Maryland to buy their booze. The high figures don't necessarily indicate that Washington residents are heavy drinkers.

The apparent per capita consumption for the United States—the average amount an American drinks—is 2.63 gallons of absolute alcohol per year. The annual per capita consumption in France is more than 6.53 gallons of absolute alcohol, while Italy's is 4.21. America probably has many more total abstainers to bring down the average, but we're a long way from a heavy per capita consumption.

What do Americans drink?

Every year, Americans consume 1.12 gallons of absolute alcohol through 2.60 gallons of distilled spirits, 1.20 gallons of absolute alcohol through 26.6 gallons of beer, and .031 gallons of absolute alcohol through 2.16 gallons of wine.

Our drinking tastes have shifted. We drink only half the amount of distilled spirits we drank 125 years ago. Then, distilled spirits accounted for 90 percent of the alcohol consumed in this country. Now, it is less than half, with beer taking up most of the slack.

How much does the average American spend on alcohol each year?

The average American spends $187.45 on alcohol each year. This represents about 3 percent of all consumption expenditures.

We, of course, spend considerably more on food, and one and a half times more on recreation. Expenditures for tobacco are about one and a half times less than those for alcohol.

Are more Americans drinking than ever before?

Yes, more Americans are drinking than ever before—there *are* more of us. Best estimates state that there are 100,000,000 Americans who drink to varying degrees. Interestingly, the proportion of drinkers to nondrinkers has risen only slightly in the last fifteen years.

Another way of visualizing it: One-third of our population above the age of fifteen does not drink alcohol at all; one-third takes alcohol occasionally; one-third drinks regularly.

How many alcoholics are there in the United States?

U.S. government studies* define alcoholism as follows:

When a person develops increased adaptation to the effects of alcohol, so that he needs increasing doses to achieve and sustain a desired effect, and shows specific signs and symptoms of withdrawal upon suddenly stopping drinking, this is considered to be alcohol dependence or addiction. Under certain circumstances and for certain periods of time that are unique for him, an alcoholic person—one who manifests the behaviors of alcohol dependence, or alcoholism—*needs* to drink, even though he may know the potential consequences of his destructive behavior.

Using this definition, the government estimates that there are between 9,000,000 and 10,000,000 alcoholics in the United

*The first Special Report on Alcohol and Health from the Secretary of HEW to the United States Congress, December 1971.

States. This represents 10 percent of the drinking population of 100,000,000, a little less than 5 percent of the country's total population.

Whatever the number, it's too large. And it doesn't need to be.

What effect did the American occupation of Japan after World War II have on Japanese drinking habits?

In my opinion, the Japanese experience strongly indicates that alcohol problems are learned, not inherited. Before World War II, the Japanese were models of responsible drinking behavior. While drinking was common, drunkenness and drinking problems were not.

During the American occupation, the Japanese people adopted many American customs, including our way of drinking. They substituted American-style cocktail bars and their ubiquitous hostesses for the civilized food, song, and drink of the geisha house. Drunkenness became common. Alcohol problems began to grow and become a concern to the Japanese people.

Why do American Indians and the Irish have a notoriously high rate of alcoholism?

The common denominator is deprivation. The American Indian was deprived of his culture, his land, his pride, his physical well-being, his dignity. He was also deprived of an opportunity to learn how to drink. In an unpracticed, physically and emotionally deprived person, small doses of alcohol produce big responses.

The Irish did have practice in drinking, but for the wrong reasons and in the wrong way. The Irish were deprived of heterosexual exposure and economic opportunity. Irish mothers approved of their boys getting drunk at the bar—it meant they weren't getting women into sexual trouble. Irish fathers didn't mind their boys getting drunk, either. In rural Ireland, the farm was the only economic resource, and it didn't necessarily go to the oldest son on the death of the father. The father could leave it to any son he wished, and he usually kept the decision to himself as long as possible so that the others would hang around working and waiting to know. Keeping drunk helped the boys bear the uncertainty.

The resulting stereotype has created, as usual, a self-fulfilling prophecy. Indians and Irish continue to have alcohol problems. An Indian said, "You see one drunk Indian, you see a thousand drunk Indians. You see one drunk white man, you only see one drunk white man." We see only one drunk white man if he isn't Irish.

Why do the French, but not the Italians, have a serious alcohol problem, when both give their children alcohol at an early age?

An Italian child is given alcohol as just another part of eating and socializing. You take food, you sip a little, you talk and laugh a little, and you don't get drunk. It's no big deal.

French children are taught that wine is the beverage of choice. Water is unsafe, and no one beyond the age of six months can comfortably digest milk. Moreover, French children see around them people who drink continuously. They grow up with this poor image of drinking habits.

Which ethnic groups in America are least likely to become alcoholic?

First-generation Italians, Jews, or Chinese are unlikely to become alcoholic. As a matter of fact, if the Italian remains within an Italian setting, if the Jew clings to his orthodoxy, or if the Chinese do not become Americanized, alcoholism is extremely rare among them.

Their children, however, become Americanized. They take up the drinking customs of the great American culture and move away from their ethnic drinking behavior. Not completely, however. Second-generation Italians and Jews do not feel kindly toward drunkenness. Alcohol for them is a part of, rather than the reason for, an activity.

By the third generation, the dilution is even greater. Getting bombed with the boys once in a while is not uncommon. Socialization with the focus on heavy drinking is usual. American drinking habits replace ethnic values. Alcoholics with Jewish and Italian and Chinese names show up in the clinics.

On the Job

In many ways, our work defines us. Our social status, our friends, even our family relationships very much depend on the work we do. Add to this the traditions, the associates, and the pressures of our working world, and it is not hard to see that our job must strongly influence our approach to alcohol.

Alcohol in business—good or bad?

Alcohol is standard equipment in American business and professional life. Take Washington, D.C., as a case in point. Socializing in Washington is an extension of office hours; only the locus changes. Information is passed, pacts are made, business relations are formed. Alcohol is often a useful catalyst in these dealings, and the social setting legitimizes its use. As a result, a lot of drinking goes on in that so-called social setting, and lunches and business dinners are heavily laced with alcohol. Certainly the Washington situation is not unique, but wherever it exists, it can become unhealthy.

Drinking can be good and useful for the socializing parts of business; but when drinking is used or needed *in order to function* in business or professionally—for instance, when you use it regularly to keep your tension level in control so you can concentrate, or use it before a difficult meeting to bolster your courage, or to relieve early-morning nerves, then you ought to exercise some caution.

If you don't want to drink as much as your business seems to require, you can find a good camouflage among the drinks listed on page 158.

Do the military services have unusual drinking problems?

Recent studies do indicate a serious misuse of alcohol and a large number of alcohol problems in the military. People in the services drink out of boredom and because it is part of the accepted stereotype of the serviceman. Activities planned as alternatives to drinking to fill free time would help. It might also be useful to discontinue the very large discount on liquor that is usual in PXs. I don't believe that raising prices for the general public will prevent people from using alcohol. But it does seem that making liquor almost as inexpensive as soda on military posts could be considered a form of pushing the drug. The implications of heavy alcohol consumption for the well-being of the people serving our country and for the military's effectiveness need to be studied.

What other fields include a lot of alcoholics?

According to the American Medical Association, alcoholism causes four hundred doctors to leave the practice of medicine each year. Considering that doctors, as highly esteemed members of the community, need to be terribly sick with alcoholism before anyone will dare notice and diagnose them, that's a lot of doctors (almost four full medical school graduating classes). And we are suffering the loss during a period when we're concerned about a shortage of physicians.

In the nineteenth century, the only major American writer popularly known to suffer a severe alcohol problem was Edgar Allan Poe. In the twentieth century, the number of writers known to have severe alcohol problems is staggering. Some may contend that the facts are easier to come by now. I believe we make inordinate demands on public figures, gobbling them up quickly in today's instant-communication world. The pressure forces many of them to the anesthetic solace of alcohol.

Why do so many people in powerful positions have drinking problems?

Power, in and of itself, is intoxicating. People who enjoy the power high tend to lean toward other intoxicating mechanisms. Drinking is a common, easily accessible one.

There are other reasons. Powerful people are constantly courted with parties and socializing and are frequently put into heavy drinking situations. Many powerful people also get into trouble with alcohol because they need heavy doses to relieve the mental and physical tensions of power.

A member of Congress once said publicly, "There is no better training ground for alcoholism than serving in the Congress of the United States." His statement does not mean we are being served in Congress only by alcoholically ill people, but that frequent and heavy drinking is an occupational hazard of a power center like the Congress.

Why do the spouses of many famous people have drinking problems?

Fame exacts a price: You must constantly live up to an image perceived by others instead of being what you really are. The substitutive reward is the ego satisfaction of adulation and recognition.

The spouse, as a mere appendage, has an even greater loss of self-perceived identity than the famed mate, and his or her satisfactions are at best vicarious. Vicarious satisfactions are poor food for the human spirit. The hunger to be recognized as an individual is quieted by heavy doses of drink. Certainly in that situation one identity is easy to achieve: Be an alcoholic.

Why do many housewives have a drinking problem?

Boredom and feeling unneeded are the enemies of sanity. Whoever and wherever we are, whatever personal terrors plague us, we divert our aloneness and anxiety by being usefully engaged and feeling wanted and needed.

There was a time when to be a housewife was an active, demanding, and needed occupation. Time and technology changed that. Now the job seems demeaning and unimportant, and women seek other outlets.

Housewives who, for whatever reasons, are not free to fly their cage increasingly depend on frequent doses of alcohol. In the reveries of heavy drink, boredom and feelings of being unneeded melt away.

Why do certain kinds of work have a higher rate of alcoholism?

The demands of the work and the nature of the exposure to alcohol are frequently at fault. Studies show that the set and circumstances under which we drink may have more to do with developing problems than individual psychological needs alone.

Certain professions are highly tension-producing, with drinking very much part of the scene. Such professions are theater, TV, magazine, and newspaper work—jobs with tight deadlines, public exposure, and the pressure to excel. Some people use alcohol as a tool in their work or social lives: salespeople and politicians, to put clients or colleagues in a more receptive mood; social climbers, to woo important people. Some jobs are boring and lonely, and the people engaged in them use alcohol to relieve their discomfort.

We do not know whether the profession causes the individual's alcohol problem or whether he or she chooses the profession that makes it easy to develop alcoholism.

What are the business advantages, if any, of drinking?

In our society there is a kind of suspicion of the nondrinker. Is he struggling with an alcohol problem? Is she a teetotaler who is going to lecture us? Is he being unfriendly? Why is he afraid to let down his controls with me? What's he hiding? The business advantage of drinking may be that of belonging and being accepted.

There is another advantage if the relationship, though necessary to business, is dull or unpleasant: drinking responsibly makes the activity tolerable.

How much money does American business lose each year due to alcoholism?

According to a recent government study, the United States loses over $25 billion annually to alcohol misuse and alcoholism. Lost production costs account for $9.5 billion; $8.25 billion is lost to health and medical costs; $6.5 billion is lost because of motor vehicle accidents; and $500 million is lost in costs to the criminal justice system. The rest of the costs are for the treatment and welfare systems.

Your Children

National attitudes, peer group standards, and personal needs will create your children's drinking patterns, just as they have created yours. But you have some influence, too. You may as well use it to help them learn to use alcohol well.

Should I teach my children to drink? What should I tell them?

If you drink, you *are* teaching your children to drink. All studies confirm that the way you drink is likely to be the way they are going to drink. A drinking parent is probably going to have drinking offspring.

We may not be aware of it, but we teach our children about alcohol very early in life. Take toddlers. They notice that Mommy and Daddy and their friends behave in a particular way. Then they notice that when the grown-ups drink this particular liquid—which is usually denied to the children, so they can't miss the fact that it's something special—then Mommy and Daddy and their friends behave differently. Anyone who has been a parent knows how children always ask to taste or have anything that you are enjoying. When it's coffee we give them a sip and laugh when they don't like it. But when it comes to alcohol, without recognizing our inconsistency, we say, "You can't have it because it's not good for you." That is one kind of education.

Part of the teaching comes from outside the home. People make a great many jokes about alcohol. A fancy dress is often called a cocktail dress. We name events after alcohol—cocktail parties, beer busts, wine-tasting parties, and so forth. Many songs are related to alcohol. People drink and get drunk on television. Our magazines are full of advertisements for alcohol. And if you can manage to get some of the powers of the liquor industry talking off the record, they will tell you that they never sell alcohol; they really sell sex and sophistication. The alcohol is merely a subliminal partner. Children pick up all these signals. That's another kind of education.

There is little that we parents can do about signals from the world at large, but for the part of the education that we can control, we should teach them by taste and example. If you're drinking and they want to have a sip, give it to them after cautioning them that they may not like the taste. Why not?

Other cultures do it. Many don't think there is anything special about giving alcohol to their young and don't even have legal drinking ages. Nobody makes a fuss about it, and these groups use alcohol without appreciable problems. We make a great deal of fuss about it, and we seem to have plenty of problems. Remove the mystery, defuse the allure of the unknown, don't set up barriers. Who struggles very hard for what they can get easily?

If children want more than they should have (an unlikely possibility), we can set the limit appropriate to their age and development. Common sense and our own intuition is still the best formula in a pinch.

As to telling children about liquor, I would give them the facts included in this book when they're ready to know. But telling is much less important than showing. The best teaching is to set an example you want them to emulate.

Do the children of alcoholic parents have a higher rate of alcoholism than the children of nonalcoholic parents?

There is little doubt that children whose parents are alcoholic are more likely than others to develop alcohol problems. A study shows that they may also be more prone to develop other behavioral problems as well. The alcohol problems can be considered as behavior *learned* from adults who were significant to the child.

One of the reasons America needs to come to grips with the safe use of alcohol as well as its problems is the contagion factor. We tend to think of contagion as referring only to disease spread through germs. But learned unhealthy, dangerous behavior is just as contagious, just as sickness-producing.

If we can spread dysfunctional and debilitating ways of living, doesn't it follow that we can transmit healthy, responsible ones as well? When more people in this country learn how to use alcohol as it should be used, all our children will have more good examples of successful drinking, and children of alcoholic parents will have better models to learn from.

Can teenagers really handle alcohol?

I know of nothing about alcohol or teenagers that would preclude their handling alcohol well. In drinking, as in most things, experience and responsibility and self-respect tend to lead to a favorable outcome. Young people haven't had time to gain much experience, so be sure that you provide favorable circumstances, preferably at home, for them to practice their drinking.

Teenagers are people. If people can handle alcohol, then I don't see why teenagers cannot. The teenagers I've studied handle alcohol about as well as the adults who were their models.

All the kids were smoking pot, but now I hear that most of them are returning to alcohol. What happened?

Pot is not a new drug. It's a natural substance like alcohol and has been around for social use almost as long as alcohol has. But it never caught on except in special circumstances—circumstances that support introspection, meditation, and isolation. Though pot smoking is often done in groups with initial community feeling, usually the individual soon drifts into an isolated reverie state. Alcohol causes most people to reach out—it is for socializing and sociability.

When adults became horrified about the use of pot among young people, we sold them on it as a symbol of their separateness from us. Young people are less interested in separateness now. The young have essentially returned to the value fold of their parents. And they've taken with them their parents' drug of choice, alcohol.

When teenagers begin to drink, why do they booze it up?

Young people approach drinking—a major rite of passage between childhood and adulthood in our society—with their usual exuberance and energy. Unpracticed drinkers that they are, they believe one has a good time with alcohol only by getting drunk. Therefore, they exaggerate the amount they've consumed and, most certainly, the effect that alcohol has on them. Young people equate boozed up with grown up. No one teaches or shows them the safe way to drink.

Boozed up, in some groups, means belonging. At that uncertain age, every ounce of belonging—even to the point of having to get drunk—is worth all the misery and risk of overdrinking.

Why do college students throw so many drunken beer parties?

The college experience, in the main, is a last fling. Those people who are fortunate enough to get to college know that they are enjoying the last years of childhood dependence. Drunken beer parties symbolize childhood's indulgence and freedom without responsibility.

Do the youth of other countries have drinking problems?

Some do. The drunkenness of some Soviet youth is called hooliganism. Swedish young people get drunk often, too. If a country's adult population has drinking problems, you can bet that a like proportion of its young do, too.

Our two teenagers drink, and we're disturbed about it; but we'd be more disturbed if they were taking drugs. Is it better not to make a fuss about it?

Your two teenagers *are* taking drugs; alcohol is a drug. I wouldn't make a fuss about it, but if you're disturbed, I'd sure discuss with them how you feel about it. Parents have an obligation to let their children know how they feel about things. If you're disturbed, you're disturbed. Tell them why you're disturbed—especially if you yourself drink.

I do think most of us parents would be more comfortable than we are about all drug use by teenagers (as well as adults) if we could separate out in our minds the big difference between use and misuse.

Everybody in my son's high school drinks. Is this typical?

According to the findings of a nationwide government study done in 1975 at randomly selected high schools, 93 percent of the boys and 87 percent of the girls have had experience with the drinking of alcohol. We'd have to conclude that drinking, or at least trying alcohol, is typical behavior among high school students.

How many teenagers in America are alcoholics? How many are misusing alcohol?

One nongovernment study estimated that there are 500,000 alcoholic teenagers in the United States. The figure may not be accurate, but even if it's only close, it's alarming.

A government study, done in 1975, was not designed to find out how many alcoholics there are, but it showed that a little more than a million young people are misusing alcohol. Misuse was measured by frequency of drunkenness and appropriateness of drinking. Five percent of the kids are overdosing with alcohol at least once a week.

But if you examine only students in the upper grades, at age seventeen, you find that 14 percent of male seniors report overdosing with alcohol—getting drunk—at least once a week.

That's bad enough, but then you take a sample a bit younger, and at the tenth-grade level you find that 50 percent of all students surveyed report drinking at night *in cars*. Now, consider the fact that, for all drivers, 40 percent of deaths on the highway are alcohol-related. But for drivers between sixteen and twenty-four, no less than 60 percent of traffic fatalities are alcohol-related.

So it's clear that alcohol is contributing to a great many youthful deaths. Go on to the possibility of present and future alcoholism with all its physical and social implications, and you can see there's a big problem that demands action. What that action should be requires serious, informed discussion, but a good starting place would be for parents to take a look at their own attitudes and drinking behavior. What are we teaching our children?

Drinking and Driving

Though your drinking always affects or is affected by other people, never does the alcohol link between you and others have more drastic implications than when you have been drinking and are at the wheel of a car.

How many drinks can I have and still drive safely?

Anstie's limit of safe drinking allows for one or two drinks. This generally brings the blood alcohol level no higher than 0.05 percent. Studies show that a drinker at the 0.05 percent level is at no greater risk of a traffic accident than the nondrinker. So, in general, it is safe to drive after one or two.

But again, statistics are not individuals. Under some circumstances even a little makes us tipsy, and we need to be alert to those times when our response to drinking is different from usual.

How much does it really take to impair my driving ability?

The average-size person quickly downing either three shots of whiskey, five eight-ounce glasses of beer, or four glasses of wine is impaired for driving. Any drinking that begins to push our blood alcohol level above the 0.05 percent mark impairs our driving. The higher the blood alcohol level, the greater the risk. By the time a blood alcohol level of 0.2 percent is reached, the risk of an accident is one hundred times that for the nondrinking driver.

Most tests given to people arrested for drunken driving in the United States show a blood alcohol level of 0.2 percent. To get an 0.2 percent level, a person would need to drink approximately ten drinks within an hour. That's a lot of determined drinking.

Aren't the breathalyzer and urine tests unfair?

The breathalyzer, even with its imperfections (a heavy dose of garlic or a case of emphysema or bronchitis causes a false reading, and false results can occasionally occur when deeply expired air is not collected), is a generally reliable approach to trying to identify drunk drivers. What's more, it's a reasonable method of showing that society disapproves of individuals who drive a car while drunk. We believe that drinking is a matter of choice but driving is a privilege that does not include the right to endanger others.

Using a urine test is unfair. Urine studies don't accurately reflect the effect of alcohol on us.

How many accidents in America are related to alcohol?

Heavy drinking and accidents show a high correlation in America. Forty percent of all traffic fatalities on the highway are alcohol-related. Among young drivers, those between the ages of sixteen and twenty-four, 60 percent of fatalities are due to heavy drinking.

Nonfatal automobile accidents are also closely related to heavy alcohol use, as are fires involving persons and property. In addition, one study showed that 58 percent of home accidents occurred as a result of drinking.

When we are heavily anesthetized with a drug, our reflexes, our judgment, and our awareness are slowed. We become accident-prone.

The Law

The law intervenes in a number of ways in the individual's use of alcohol. Attempts at prevention and punishment have been largely ineffective, but when misuse by any individual threatens the safety of others, the law quite rightly steps in.

Why can't minors drink? Can they drink at home?

By law, we limit the age at which persons can purchase and consume alcoholic beverages in public places. The age ranges from eighteen to twenty-one, but since studies show that most young people take alcohol much before the age of eighteen, these laws are largely ineffectual.

Minors can drink in their own homes, presumably with parental permission. I don't believe the police will interfere if your liquor supply is used by your child, even without your permission. They will interfere in certain locales, however, if alcohol is served to someone else's minor child without the parent's permission.

In setting drinking ages, the law serves one questionable purpose: It increases the lure of the forbidden surrounding alcohol. When a person reaches his or her majority at eighteen and can engage in all adult activities with the exception of buying and consuming drinks, alcohol has been put in an exalted position that it does not deserve.

While I was still teaching at Harvard, I remember students telling me what fun it was when they were nineteen and twenty (the legal drinking age was then twenty-one in Massachusetts) to get a supply of liquor and get bombed. But then they'd find themselves in the neighboring state of New York where the legal age was eighteen. They'd walk in and order a drink. Often they didn't care to finish it. With the removal of the barriers, the fun and interest were gone.

Since alcoholism is our number-one drug problem, why isn't alcohol, like heroin, outlawed?

Until recent years, heroin was mainly a drug of the deprived. But when young people, especially those of the rock culture, began to find it fashionable to behave as though they were deprived, the use of heroin spread. Heroin is very addictive and should be avoided, but our real reason for outlawing it is that it's unfamiliar. It is not the social drug of most people. Alcohol is. We are therefore incensed about the heroin problem and spend huge sums of money to solve it, but scarcely notice the far greater destruction resulting from the misuse of our favored drug.

If laws were passed making booze more costly and more difficult to find, would this reduce the number of drunks?

The Canadian government, acting on the assumption that reducing consumption will reduce drunkenness, is considering a policy of severely limiting liquor licenses and advertising, as well as imposing high taxes on liquor. My colleagues and I have argued about this approach, and some of us are convinced it is wrong. Greater cost means that rich drunks will pay more to get drunk. Greater cost means that poor drunks will get poorer getting drunk or seek cheaper (possibly dangerous) forms of alcohol. The moderate drinker, on the other hand, may give up this pleasure as too costly. But is it the moderate drinker we are trying to dissuade? Do we want our only model of the drinker to be the drunk?

As to making alcohol less readily available—some years ago when Nikita Khrushchev was still in power, the Soviets, alarmed over drunkenness, decided to limit the sale of vodka to one drink in a bar. They reasoned that, since the bars were far apart, the drinker would have metabolized his vodka by the time he reached the next saloon to buy his single shot. In a sense, it worked. Vodka sales went down. The manufacture of home brew, however, shot up, and Russian drunkenness remained.

The ingenuity that people will exercise to get what they feel they want and need is remarkable. And the ones who suffer from regulations designed to control behavior are those who are least likely to be misbehaving in the first place.

Should we legislate drinking behavior?

To try to legislate behavior is foolish. Better to let drunkenness go the way of spitting—once a popular American pastime. Spitting was made a punishable offense, but the law was not what ended it. It's no longer popular in America because people no longer approve of it—it fell out of favor.

The same thing can happen to drunkenness—unless we try to forbid it by law. The reason many of us began to drink and tried to tie one on in the first place was that it was taboo. That's why lots of young people drink in cars or parking lots or basements, chewing on mints, hoping the smell and taste will go away. I suspect that every law we pass making it difficult or guilt-producing to drink only makes us drink more.

Why is absinthe outlawed?

Absinthe is a liqueur of high alcohol content (136 proof) that was the first alcoholic drink singled out for total prohibition. In 1905 in Switzerland a husband, "temporarily blinded with rage from drinking absinthe," brutally shot and murdered his wife and children. The country was so incensed by this act that within two years the manufacture, sale, and importation of absinthe was barred in Switzerland.

In spite of this horrible event and the conclusion of a psychiatric witness at the trial that "absinthe created an irresistible temptation to drink more," Ernest Hemingway and others extolled its virtues. They raved about absinthe as an aphrodisiac—the best and safest. The best and safest "because its action changed ideas instead of stimulating sexual glands as do most aphrodisiacs," said Hemingway in *For Whom the Bell Tolls*.

We purportedly did not ban absinthe because of its "irresistible," "sexual," and "assaultive" potential. Absinthe contains extractions of wormwood, which has a high content of thujone, a highly toxic substance. Our law says that alcohol must be almost 100 percent thujone-free, and we allow only vermouth, with minor quantities of thujone, to be consumed.

Alcoholism

A great many Americans drink sensibly, and with some new understandings and attitudes many more could do as well. But alcohol abuse has been and continues to be a very major problem for many of us. Sensible drinking is one thing, as we've seen; alcoholism is another.

When we talk about alcoholism

Information and openness are as important in discussing alcoholism as they are when we discuss sensible drinking. We can save ourselves, our friends, families, and colleagues a great deal of grief if we're willing to become informed about how and why many people deprive themselves of the benefits of moderate drinking.

There are, of course, many kinds of pain from which people seek relief in the anesthetic effect of alcohol. Some of these people will abuse alcohol for a limited time only. Others may seek its release so continuously that the alcohol becomes more destructive than the pain it was intended to relieve.

Whether drinking turns into abuse or abuse into alcoholism depends as much on society as it does on the individual drinker. A society's prevailing attitude toward alcohol shapes the drinking habits of all its members; so in order to understand why a large segment of our society makes alcohol—a useful drug—into a problem drug, let's look again at our attitudes about alcohol and those who abuse it.

In America we are not only uptight and preoccupied about alcohol, we are vindictive and punitive toward alcoholics. These attitudes surface in a number of ways: (1) paternalism, or talking down to; (2) impossible standards of recovery (no drink ever, so that failure is almost guaranteed); and (3) a kind of therapeutic nihilism (diagnosis and treatment are both hard to get). At almost every level of society there is a negative feeling for people who, we feel, are having a good time losing control with alcohol while we have to behave ourselves.

Nothing, of course, could be farther from the truth. Alcoholic people don't really enjoy alcohol—they need the relief it brings. The society that screams at them, and laments them, seems not to understand how desperate a person must be to choose—if he does, in fact, choose—an illness so despised by the rest of us.

What is alcoholism?

To focus only on the alcohol in the definition of alcoholism is, I think, missing the point. All illness is socioculturally determined. There is no biologically labeled illness. Illness is what we label it, whether it is physical, psychological, or cultural. For example, suppose there existed a remote island where the people had lost contact with the rest of the world. Suppose they had been in the path of one of the first hydrogen bombs and through genetic malformation everyone now alive there had only one leg. If you or I were suddenly transported to that island, we would be "deviants," the ill ones, because we have two legs.

When do you get sick? You "get sick" when you're diagnosed, which means that either you saw something different or dysfunctional about yourself, or society said there was something different and dysfunctional. Imagine a person with the delusion of being Christ reincarnated. He is not troubled by it, and he shows no external signs of the delusion. Is he "sick"? Imagine an autopsy after an automobile accident. The pathologist finds an asymptomatic malignancy. The person did not know there was a malignancy, and society did not know. (The tumor, as sometimes happens, was getting better all by itself.) So, was the person "sick"?

This idea applies to alcohol problems. If you are preoccupied with alcohol, if you or others in your environment are discomfited by this preoccupation, if alcohol interferes with your ability to function in other necessary ways, then you are suffering from alcoholism.

Is alcoholism an illness, or is it a bad habit that's hard to break?

Alcoholism is an illness. It's not a bad habit. When we can't reach an alcoholic we care about, we sometimes get so frustrated that we convince ourselves he's bad, and not sick.

Think about it for a minute. Can we believe that anyone, given an alternative way to relieve the pain he or she is anesthetizing with alcohol, would want to be an alcoholic? I've never met anyone who would. That is not to say, though, that we don't need to reinforce the individual's underlying desire to recover. Society's disdain, disgust, and disrespect for alcoholic people makes them less willing to recognize their problem and seek help. The scarlet "A" of the twentieth century is no great pleasure to wear.

Is it true that some people can become alcoholics from the first drink?

People always ask, "What about the person who takes one drink and is a confirmed alcoholic?" I have heard these stories, too, and a few patients have reported that this was their history. But I also know that if an Orthodox Jewish rabbi were eating some meat and you informed him it was meat from a pig, he would have a physiological response. The rabbi would probably feel nauseated. He might even vomit. Yet I can't conceive that there is a metabolic defect in Orthodox Jews that causes a reaction to pork products. So, yes, I can imagine certain combinations of physical, psychological, and cultural experiences that could produce an unusual response to the first drink—a response that could label someone as an alcoholic from the first drink. But it wouldn't be the alcohol that did it, and such a response would be very rare indeed.

I remember all too vividly the tragic story of one patient who had been born illegitimately and abandoned in a public toilet. This was something she never could get over—she spoke of it often, really thought of herself as a piece of feces, and thought that until she died. She was put into a boarding home for a time and was then reclaimed by her mother. When she was eight, her mother made some home brew and put it in the refrigerator, and my patient and her stepsister stealthily tasted it. The sister immediately became ill—she could not stand the stuff. But my patient kept drinking it until she fell unconscious, and she drank in that pattern all of her life. I think she could be considered an alcoholic from her first drink.

Are alcoholics always alcoholics?

Most recovered alcoholics say they are. They say it with pride for having recovered and as a reminder that they think alcohol is still a danger to them. I suspect that there's nothing wrong with their position. My concern is that an illness not become the identity of a person.

I'm uncomfortable when a person is called a diabetic or a cardiac. People are dehumanized when they're labeled by a condition.

Should I drink in the presence of a recovered alcoholic?

Why not? If we don't, someone else is sure to. We're a drinking society. If recovered alcoholic people want to avoid drinking people, they'll need to get on the next moon shot.

As a matter of fact, recovered alcoholic people are uncomfortable if they think you want to drink but refrain out of deference to their illness.

They consider it a putdown, evidence that you consider them weak and in need of protection.

Am I correct in thinking that alcoholics are people who function at a low level and who, if cured, would not be of much benefit to society?

Baloney! If it were not for alcoholic people, both recovered and unrecovered, a great many beautiful contributions to the world would not exist. Alcoholics are people like you and me. Like most illnesses, alcoholism recognizes no economic, racial, or age boundaries—young and old, black and white, rich and poor, dropouts and Ph.D.s are all potential victims.

Can a recovered alcoholic ever drink socially?

There is abundant evidence that even some severe alcoholics go back to social drinking, although why they'd run the risk is beyond me. Alcohol is no necessity of life. Alcoholism can rob us of life. Social drinking after severe alcoholism isn't such a good idea.

Some alcoholics dare not touch a drop, but there are lots of people with less severe alcoholism or alcohol problems who can drink socially after treatment. We need to make these distinctions.

Too many people don't go for treatment because they can't imagine making a commitment to a dry state forever. If they're reminded that no decision is for always, they'll come to treatment sooner. After all, these days, even deciding to get married doesn't seem to mean you're deciding forever.

But remember that the studies that conclude that recovered alcoholics can drink socially are reports based on statistical averages. The average will include some who encounter no difficulty, some who have an occasional mild relapse, and some who relapse into alcoholism completely. We have to be very careful about applying broad findings based on a statistical average to specific individuals. They obviously don't apply to everyone, and can be dangerously wrong for some.

Why do we condone drunkenness but not alcoholism?

Getting drunk is a temporary but familiar experience. We do not pay it much mind. We really sanction it.

We sanction it as we do beating the income tax and shady business deals—they're all right as long as they're not exposed and prosecuted. When the law moves in and labels the person involved a criminal, however, we turn on him.

The same is true of alcohol. Many a heavy drinker commands respect and admiration, even on those occasions when he's loaded. But let that same person—perhaps even with the same drinking pattern and prowess—be labeled alcoholic, and we feel contempt or possibly condescension toward him. Temporary lapses are tolerated. The permanence implied by the diagnosis of alcoholism is another matter.

We forget that when we tolerate the one, the other tags along—in time—behind.

If there are 10,000,000 alcoholics in America, how come I don't notice them?

It is human nature not to see what we do not wish to see. I know that my special interest in alcoholism means that I'm sensitive to clues and that people, once they realize that I am not going to judge them, tend to tell me about alcoholic problems in themselves, their families, or among their friends. No matter where I go the problem appears or is discussed. But that isn't the experience of most people. Besides, because alcoholism is stigmatized, it is very carefully hidden.

What causes alcoholism? The alcohol or the person?

For centuries, the focus was on the substance—alcohol. The belief that alcohol caused alcoholism was reinforced when specific organisms (for example, the tubercle bacillus in tuberculosis) were found to be related to the cause of some diseases. Since in Western societies the prevailing belief has been that human beings are basically weak-willed, it followed that exposure to the temptation of alcohol would inevitably lead to alcoholism. And the reverse, of course, was true: Without alcohol there would be no alcoholism. Equally true: Without a tubercle bacillus, there would be no tuberculosis. And yet in both conditions (alcoholism and tuberculosis), exposure is unrelated to illness.

Most people have the tubercle bacillus within them and have not developed active tuberculosis. Most people drink and do not become alcoholic. This obvious fact shifted the focus, in a large way, to the person. What makes a person vulnerable? There are all kinds of theories—entire books have been written about the causes.

I believe that if you mix the pharmacologic action of alcohol, a person in physical, psychological, or social pain, and a society that is ambivalent, conflicted, and guilty about its use of alcohol, you have a working answer.

We know alcohol is a readily available anesthetic agent effective in temporarily relieving all types of pain, and that pain (from whatever origin) cries out for relief. We know a society's confusion over a substance often results in overemphasizing its value. But we might ask: In America we're all exposed to the unhealthy focus on drinking, we all have alcohol, we all have pain—why do some people become alcoholics, while the vast majority do not?

Usually the added ingredient is being influenced by someone, often during the formative years, who set the model for solving problems with alcohol. Among two-thirds of all alcoholics, the model was someone very close.

Again, in this as other general observations, there are exceptions. And with some alcoholics it's hard to pinpoint the cause or causes of the problem.

Alcoholism: Diagnosis

People in the field of alcohol abuse can debate endlessly the fine lines of distinction among the varying degrees of abuse. Here, for better or worse, are mine.

Define alcoholism

Alcoholism is a severe chronic preoccupation with, or use of, alcohol that interferes with the person's ability to function in his or her normal way at work, at home, or with friends. Many persons with alcoholism are physically addicted to alcohol.

How do alcohol abuse, alcoholism, and a drinking problem differ?

Every time we get drunk or drink more than Anstie's limit, we've experienced alcohol abuse. It doesn't mean we need to be diagnosed or treated. It is a sign that something was wrong when we drank.

Alcoholism is farther down the road of abuse. The overuse is consistent and frequent, of great intensity, and it overwhelms most of the rest of our life's interests and activities. There is a strong possibility of developing a physical addiction.

A drinking problem lies between alcohol abuse and alcoholism. Any alcohol problem, mild or severe, greatly increases our chances for becoming alcoholic.

What are the signs of a drinking problem?

1. Frequent episodes of drunkenness (more than four times in one year).
2. Needing alcohol to cope with fears, relieve everyday pressures, or escape loneliness.
3. Needing alcohol to be able to do whatever daily tasks confront us.
4. Frequent hangovers, dizziness, or physical discomfort.
5. Accidents while drinking: in a car, at home, and so on.
6. Difficulties with work as a consequence of drinking.

7. Difficulties with home or social life as a consequence of drinking.
8. A marked personality change while drinking.
9. Behaving when under the influence of alcohol in ways we contend we'd never behave had we been sober.
10. Blackouts.
11. Memory lapses.

When is someone a heavy drinker?

A heavy drinker is usually a person who consumes more than Anstie's limit of safe drinking.

My husband says he's just a social beer drinker, but every time he goes out drinking, he comes home drunk. He insists he doesn't have a drinking problem because he often goes for weeks without taking a drink. Does he have a drinking problem?

He surely does. Getting drunk every time one drinks—no matter how little or how much is consumed—is a true indication that a drinking problem exists. Many problem drinkers are spree drinkers. Even the most severely ill alcoholic people have periods when they do not drink.

What about someone like me? I don't get drunk, but I need a drink to function.

If alcohol is the fuel to get your human engine running, you've got an engine in need of repair. When we're dependent on alcohol to function, we've definitely got a drinking problem.

Treatment

There is no single treatment now known that is effective for every alcoholic, and there is evidence to suggest that more people would seek treatment if some less rigid or less demanding approaches were introduced.

If I want to recover from alcoholism, what are my chances?

The chances are superb. Two out of three people recover. Those who don't make it the first time ought not to quit trying. There are different treatments for different people. If a given treatment program doesn't work after a good try, it doesn't mean we're untreatable. It only means it was not the right program for us.

Seventy percent of the alcoholic people who receive treatment in federally funded alcohol programs recover; that is, they can resume normal functioning. Recovery rates are similar for nonfederally funded programs. (This happens in spite of doctors' not diagnosing until very late, in spite of unrealistic success criteria, and in spite of physicians who don't know much about the problem.) Alcoholics Anonymous is a highly successful treatment program. Business and industry alcoholism programs that make early identification of alcohol problems in employees have even higher success rates.

Is there a cure?

For far too long we have condemned alcoholic people to the prison of unrealistic expectations. There may not be cure (that is, a return to the pre-illness state), but there is plenty of healthy and useful recovery.

Success is there for anyone who cares to see it, and yet the prevailing attitude is that alcoholic people don't do well in treatment. This false notion is the result of unrealistic expectations. Let me give you an example.

A colleague once remarked that people were disappointed in the psychiatric treatment of depression. They thought that the treated person would never get depressed again. That's a pretty unrealistic expectation in view of the state of the world.

People have the same kinds of expectations for the alcoholic's recovery. He's not allowed any relapses or slips. But who goes through life without setbacks? And when we do experience setbacks, it's quite common for us to return to patterns of coping that are familiar or have brought us relief in the past. I am not surprised that a person with a long history of problems with alcohol regresses to the solace of alcoholic anesthesia in the face of some overwhelming stress and pain. But our demands are so high, and we make alcoholics feel so guilty and lost if they slip, that the slip often turns into a total relapse.

Instead of celebrating whatever period of self-respect, dignity, and functioning the alcoholic person enjoys, we signal our feeling of pessimism about his or her recovery. We wait—as we force the person to do—with bated breath for a relapse. Then our prophecy is fulfilled.

A rheumatologist thinks he's doing very well if his arthritic patient is pain-free and functioning for six months or longer. Other specialists, too, are grateful for less than perfect, permanent cure. Those treating alcoholics should offer a realistic helping hand, aiming for cure but happy with good periods of recovery.

Where can I go for help?

Anyone with an alcohol problem can contact the alcoholism agency in each state to find out where to go for help. Appendix V contains a complete listing of state agencies, with addresses and phone numbers.

The National Council on Alcoholism has affiliated groups in most localities that can refer people to appropriate treatment resources. In the telephone book the name of the city in which the affiliate exists precedes the council's name; for example, Washington Area Council on Alcoholism, Boston Council on Alcoholism, and so on.

Alcoholics Anonymous (AA) has chapters all over. They'll help you get to an AA group, or to other treatment opportunities. They're listed in the telephone directory under Alcoholics Anonymous.

Treatment is just an inquiry away.

Why does AA work so well?

That remarkable organization, AA, works because its founders understood people and their suffering. Since all are alcoholic, AA members cannot make judgments. They offer each other acceptance and support. They reach out. They care. They understand.

The movement is modeled on the age-old, very human way of handling all kinds of afflictions. It is an extended family; it is a small community's support. And it is so obvious.

Early in my career, after my first lecture, I looked disappointed enough for my chief to ask what was troubling me. I said I was disappointed because in my lecture all I had done was state the obvious. He told me, "Morris, your entire career will be devoted to nothing more than stating the obvious."

We need to be reminded, all of us, that great therapy lies in the reaching out of one person toward another.

What's wrong with AA?

Remarkable as AA is, it's not for everyone. There are those of us who are private people and abhor the exposure that AA requires. Others have other needs.

AA has not been willing in the past (it is improving) to understand that some people need more than just AA, or not even AA. The pressures are now immense to join if you are alcoholic—recovered or not.

I recently heard of a well-known person who had recovered from alcoholism without AA. He had been making a name for himself in the alcoholism community but was not looked upon with complete favor because he had not made it through AA. Ten years after his recovery, he began to feel he wouldn't have all the credentials to be effective in the field unless he was a member of AA. So he joined.

AA creates another problem, through no fault of its own. It gives doctors an excuse to avoid learning about and dealing with alcoholics. It's easier to let AA do it.

If alcoholism is an illness, why don't doctors and hospitals treat it?

Doctors and hospitals are not terribly interested in treating alcoholic people. Our society neither knows much about alcoholism nor is it fully convinced that alcoholic people are really sick. All of us are empathic and caring if we believe people have come to grief through no fault of their own. Since most of us drink and don't have problems, we feel that alcoholic people have brought their problems on themselves. They got hooked on pleasure and became alcoholic.

Consequently, hardworking doctors in overcrowded hospitals prefer to devote their energies to more "deserving" patients whose illnesses they understand. Acceptance of the prevailing image of *the* alcoholic as a skid row person (they make up only 3 to 5 percent of the alcoholic population in this country) doesn't increase their interest.

Things are changing now. Since the profession of medicine is losing four hundred doctors every year to alcoholism, and since from 25 to 50 percent of the general hospital beds are occupied by patients whose ailments are complicated by alcohol problems, the medical profession and hospitals are waking up.

Blue Cross is moving into the picture by extending benefits to alcoholic people. Things are finally changing—and for the better!

What can the medical profession do to improve the treatment of alcoholics?

A number of studies have revealed that though physicians do give lip service to the fact that anyone can develop an alcohol problem, essentially they use the skid row derelict model for diagnosis. It's as though we diagnosed cancer only after it had metastasized through the entire body.

Our studies further reveal that one reason many physicians diagnose in this way is that they are just like the rest of us: They are more comfortable viewing the alcoholic person as someone very far out, different from themselves. By diagnosing only after the patient has dramatic symptoms, physicians avoid the need to face their own conflicts about the use of alcohol, or their own drinking habits.

Doctors can begin to improve treatment by examining their attitudes toward alcoholics. The all-American attitudes shared by most physicians affect the treatment of alcoholic persons in at least one important way. There are two general groups of people who are sensitive to real messages: the young and the sick; the young because they have not yet developed the defenses of socializing and sophistication, and the sick because they hurt so. Both groups hear the messages behind the words.

I participated in a very solid study at Harvard that confirmed that alcoholic people responded, not to the words the treatment clinician used, but to the sound of his voice. There was no correlation between what was said and the patients' responses. If the doctor sounded angry, patients did not stay on their regimes. If the doctor sounded stiff, or "professional," patients did not respond to treatment. But if the doctor sounded a little anxious and nervous, patients responded well and did as they were told. The alcoholic patients took nervousness as a sign of caring about them.

Medical schools can help by offering training in the treatment of alcoholism. Most physicians in the United States know next to nothing about the problem. They know something about the complications—that the liver or the esophagus or the pancreas goes bad as a consequence of alcohol abuse—but they don't know anything about alcohol problems, diagnosis, or treatment. It's a bit like sex—twenty years ago, almost no medical schools taught much about sexual functioning. We still don't teach our future doctors very much about alcoholism.

Can you help a problem drinker who insists he doesn't have a problem?

Yes, by sharing your concern about the effects of alcohol on him without anger, judgment, or nagging. Alcoholic people know that there is something different about their response to alcohol. They deny it to us because of *us*. We think—and they think—that there is shame and disgrace in suffering an alcohol problem. In the face of this stigma, they can't be blamed for denying their problem. In the past, when other illnesses were stigmatized, they were denied; but once the stigma was removed, the victims came forth unashamedly.

As long as alcoholics are looked upon with disgust, disdain, and disrespect, who would rush to be so labeled?

Like everyone else, alcoholic people respond to compassion, caring, and understanding. When an alcoholic can feel your honest empathy, the need to deny will melt away. Then you can help.

Is it possible to suffer from alcoholism and get by? Does it always need to be treated? Will it eventually affect my ability to function?

Of course it's possible to be an alcoholic and get by. Lots do. And it doesn't always need to be treated. There are reported cases of spontaneous recovery from alcoholism, but my guess is that someone or something outside of the person provided the shove toward recovery.

Alcoholism unchecked will in all likelihood affect a person's ability to function.

What is Antabuse? Is it a drug that cures alcoholism?

Antabuse is a drug, originated in Denmark in the late 1940s, that interferes with the usual metabolism of alcohol. Alcohol produces a toxic substance, acetylaldehyde, when it is being metabolized in our bodies. Fortunately for us, acetylaldehyde is present only moments before it is further broken down into manageable products. Antabuse maintains for just a brief moment longer than usual the presence of acetylaldehyde. That makes us damn sick. We turn lobster red, have trouble breathing, develop a severe headache, suffer nausea, and often vomit.

An alcohol-Antabuse reaction is frightening, uncomfortable, and sometimes fatal.

Antabuse is no cure for alcoholism. It must be taken daily, and missing the pill for several days allows us to drink again without a reaction. Antabuse is best prescribed for those of us who begin to drink impulsively or even automatically under given conditions. The seventy-two hours to a week needed to clear the system of Antabuse delays the impulsive response and gives us time to reach for help other than alcohol.

Antabuse should always be used as a part of a total treatment program, never as the single form of treatment. It should never be administered without the patient's knowledge.

Psychologists claim a 68 percent cure rate for neurosis. Reportedly, the cure rate for alcoholism is 70 percent. Is this a coincidence?

I don't believe a cure rate of that size for either one. I do believe that people can recover from either disability—hurt less and function better—to those percentages. I know it for sure about alcoholism. I suspect it's accurate for neurosis. It's not a coincidence. It proves a point.

People will get better—will improve and recover—when they are offered caring, compassion, and understanding. Look how many ills the old-time general practitioner cured when that's essentially all he had in his medicine bag.

Prevention

It has been said that if we were able to devise a way to detect the early warnings of cancer, perhaps 95 percent of incipient cancers could be arrested or cured. We already *know* the warning signs for developing alcohol problems. If we were able to recognize them and learn how to act on the knowledge effectively, much of the misery that alcoholism brings could be prevented.

How can alcoholism be prevented?

It will not be prevented, I am sure, by a simple vaccine or a magic formula. It doesn't have a single cause, so it will not have a single cure or a single preventive.

There are two steps toward preventing alcoholism as I define it. First, as a society, we need to establish a consensus on what the upper limits are of how, where, when, and how much we drink. When sensible, beneficial limits are established as the norm, people will be less likely to turn to overusing alcohol to solve their life problems.

This would require a profound change of value and behavior, but I believe it can be accomplished through enlightened education, inspiring national leadership, and concerned community organization. If you have doubts about the potential for change in our society, recall how, twenty-five years ago, a famous movie star's career was destroyed because she conceived a child out of wedlock, or how a film was banned because too much cleavage showed. Compare the public reaction then with today's attitudes. Change can happen. We *can* set new standards.

A sound consensus on limits sets the stage for the next step in prevention. It would make it easier to spot people who are using alcohol poorly and to offer help before severe alcoholism develops.

The truism of all health and social issues will operate: The earlier in its course a problem is diagnosed and treated, the greater the success and the lower the cost.

Right now in our personal lives and in society, we operate as firefighters who cannot smell the smoke or see the fire of impending alcoholism until it becomes a blazing inferno.

**I enjoy drinking, so I don't want to quit.
How can I be sure I won't become an alcoholic?**

You can be sure, up to a point, by following the steps of safe drinking given on pages 154–157, and by paying attention to the purpose and pattern of your drinking.

What does alcohol do for you? Is your response bizarre or unusual? Do you *need* alcohol to function? Look closely, heed what you see, and if a problem is developing, you can do something about it.

I cannot guarantee—absolutely—that you'll not become an alcoholic, but surely you will be much less likely to.

Has prohibition of alcohol ever succeeded?

Not really. Even under totalitarian regimes, attempts at prohibition have failed. The Koran forbids drinking, and yet the first Pan-Arabic Alcoholism Conference was held recently. I did meet one gentleman from a small state in India at an international meeting of world prohibitionists in Kabul, Afghanistan, who assured me that prohibition was working in his state. I cannot dispute him, but it would be a first.

What is society's role in prevention?

A subject so complex and of such broad implications demands a book of its own and goes beyond the purpose of this one. Indeed, a truly effective national approach to prevention goes far beyond education, informative pamphlets, and clever slogans, and requires us to examine our national values and in some instances to try to alter the social environment in which we live.

We need to think about the ways business and industry contribute to loneliness and anxiety. Must employees be uprooted again and again from their homes? Can workers be helped to see the worth of their individual contribution?

We must examine the drinking models provided by the media. If smoking has been largely removed from the TV screen (remember when "lighting up" was always used for dramatic emphasis, or to fill time, or to give the actor something to do with his hands?), why can't drinking of the wrong kind be eliminated, too? Why does the hero or heroine have to be shown taking a drink to brace for, or recover from, a crisis? Recently produced TV material rarely shows a performer smoking (talk shows are the exception). A little pressure from the viewers could change the quality of the drinking scenes, too.

To move to a deeper level, do the national strivings for bigness, more, and still more, create a tense and worried population? What can we do about it as individuals or as part of a group?

What are we teaching our children about drinking by our example?

The questions are difficult, the list is long, but Americans can and have produced many beneficial changes in their lives, and I believe they can do it again. The bits and pieces of change that can be brought about by individual and community action based on understanding and really caring about human needs can add up to the big changes that can prevent alcohol abuse.

Personal Drinking Records

There is a safe way to drink, and the purpose of this book is to tell you what it is. The safe limit described is a good goal to aim for, but I know most people cannot stay within it all of the time. If you think you are falling too short of the mark, a personal drinking record may give you some clues as to what is going wrong and how you can improve.

A drinking record you can use

A typical drinking record is shown in Table 1. You can see that it is a simple, straightforward, and quick way to record a time of drinking, how long it lasted (the end time), where the drinking occurred, who was there, how you were feeling, some notes about the occasion, and the reason for drinking. It is helpful to include, as a matter of course, data about the quantity and type of beverage that you consume.

Let's say, for example, that you went out with several other people and had a beer at lunch. This would be listed as one drink, the type would be beer, the occasion would be business luncheon, informal, and the three people who were with you would be listed. In addition, you would list how you relate to them; for example, your boss and two co-workers. You might also indicate how typical that was of, say, an average day or an average week. Later that evening, waiting to take the train home, you stop in a bar at the station. There you have a gin and tonic and some casual conversation with someone at the bar. This is listed on the record as a separate drinking event. After you get home, you have a martini before dinner. By this time you are relaxed and somewhat exhausted, and you record these feelings on the drinking record. You then go outside and throw a baseball around with your son and come in and have wine with your dinner. This again is recorded as a separate drinking event, including the two glasses of wine.

I suggest trying to keep this kind of daily record over a total of several typical weeks in your life. You may be quite surprised by the results. As you look them over, you might think about your priorities—what you want to get out of your own life. Is alcohol contributing to them? Is it enhancing your enjoyment of the situations you want to get the most out of?

If you decide to change some things, it is a very simple matter to keep a record for another few weeks to see whether or not you've actually succeeded.

The drinking record is more than a clever trick. Based on the

Time or Duration of Drinking Event	Place Where Event Occurred	Who Were You With?	How Were You Feeling?	Occasion and Reason for Drinking Event	Quantity and Type of Beverage Consumed	Was This Behavior Typical or Unusual for You?
Monday 1:00–2:00 P.M.	Restaurant	Boss and 2 co-workers	Relaxed	Business luncheon	1 beer	Typical
Monday 5:00–5:30 P.M.	Train-station bar	Woman at the bar	Tired	Waiting for train	1 gin and tonic	Typical
Monday 6:30–7:00 P.M.	Home	Wife	Relaxed, tired	Before-dinner drink	1 martini	Typical
Monday 7:30–9:00 P.M.	Home	Wife and son	Relaxed	Dinner	2 glasses of wine	Typical

Table 1

successful techniques of behavior therapy, it is a behavior reinforcer that gives you immediate feedback about what you are doing. It can be kept entirely private and personal, so that it is possible to modify behavior without involving others.

A couple of final notes: What should you do if you try to cut down your drinking and find that you are not doing very well? Perhaps your behavior is more ingrained than you thought. In that case, you may need stronger feedback than the drinking record can provide. I would strongly suggest that you think about the possibility that you have a drinking problem. As I said earlier, no one should go without help for a drinking problem. You deserve it, and you can get it. You need not feel guilty if you don't live up to your own expectations or if you find that you cannot always control your behavior. Think how many people in this world know smoking is bad for them, but how few have ever been able to give it up for any length of time—without help.

Suppose we expand the "drinking diary" to include several more items. In this scheme, you set up a list of your personal goals. In the next column, lay out the approximate proportion of your income that goes toward general areas that reach each of these goals. A typical example shows a person spending 26 percent on food, 24 percent on rent, 10 percent on transportation, 1 percent on books, and so on. How much is the person spending on alcohol? Again, you may be surprised. A liquor bill of several hundred dollars a month is not at all unusual, even for families with incomes between $1,000 and $1,500 a month.

Still another example of how this kind of drinking diary may work is called the "organization game." Here, once again, you list your personal goals. Beside this, have a column for the various organizations that you belong to and how actively you participate in them. In still another column, list the primary values of the people who are in these groups, including their attitudes toward drinking/nondrinking and acceptable drinking behavior. In the column next to this one, use a very simple self-rating scheme. Mark a 3 next to the organization if it is heavily focused on alcohol, 2 if it is moderately focused on alcohol, 1 if it has a very limited (but some) focus on alcohol, and 0 if it is not focused on alcohol at all. Put down a number for each of the organizations, being as honest and objective as you can. At the bottom of the column, take a simple average of the numbers. An overall average score of 2.5 would mean that most activities are rather heavily centered around alcohol. If you score higher, you should carefully consider whether you want to spend most of your time focusing on alcohol. We are not suggesting that this is psychological testing nor that it is scientific. On the other hand, it can be viewed as quite a serious "drinking game."

Sample drinking diaries

Here are some drinking diaries for you to study. Take a look at them and try to determine what your feelings and thoughts are about what role alcohol plays in the lives of these individuals.

Try to imagine who these people are and what their lives are like.

Drinking Diary 1

Day of Week	Time of Drinking	Where	Occasion	Number and Type of Drinks	Number and Type of Companions	Foods—Snacks, etc.
Monday	6:00–7:30 P.M.	Home	Cocktails	2 martinis	Wife had sherry	None
Monday	7:30–8:30 P.M.	Home	Dinner	2 glasses beer	Wife had glass wine	Full meal
Tuesday	11:30 A.M.–1:30 P.M.	Restaurant	Lunch	1 martini and 1/3 bottle wine	2 business associates	Hot lunch
Wednesday	6:00–8:00 P.M.	Bar	Cocktail—business trip	3 martinis	Alone	Chips
Wednesday	8:00–9:30 P.M.	Restaurant	Dinner	1/2 bottle wine	Alone	Full meal
Thursday	1:00–3:30 P.M.	Restaurant	Lunch	2 martinis, 2 glasses wine, 1 brandy	4 business associates, all drinking	Full meal
Thursday	6:00–8:00 P.M.	Airline	Flight home	2 martinis, 1 glass wine	Alone	Dinner
Friday	7:00 P.M.–2:00 A.M.	Friend's home	Dinner party	2 martinis, 10 glasses punch, 3 bottles beer	Wife and several other couples	Buffet
Saturday	5:30–6:30 P.M.	Home	Supper	2 bottles beer	Wife not drinking	Full meal
Sunday	2:00–6:00 P.M.	Relatives' home	Visiting in-laws	3 gin and tonics	Wife and in-laws	Full meal

Drinking Diary 2

Day of Week	Time of Drinking	Where	Occasion	Number and Type of Drinks	Number and Type of Companions	Foods—Snacks, etc.
Monday	6:00–7:00 P.M.	Home	Before dinner	1 martini	Wife drinking	None
Tuesday	12:30–2:00 P.M.	Restaurant	Business lunch	1 martini, 1 glass wine, 1 cognac	2 business associates	Full meal
Tuesday	8:00–10:30 P.M.	Home	TV—relax	2 beers	Son drinking beer	Chips
Wednesday	7:00–9:30 P.M.	Restaurant	Dinner	1 martini, ½ bottle wine, 1 cognac	Wife and another couple	Full meal
Thursday	None					
Friday	4:30–6:00 P.M.	Bar	Cocktail	3 martinis	Work associates	Snacks
Friday	7:00–9:00 P.M.	Home	Dinner	2 beers	Wife and sons	Full meal
Saturday	4:00–4:30 P.M.	Campsite	After hiking	1 beer	Wife and sons	Chips
Saturday	5:00–6:00 P.M.	Campsite	Supper	1 beer	Wife and sons	Full meal
Saturday	7:00–10:00 P.M.	Campsite	Relaxing	3 beers	Wife and sons	Snacks
Sunday	noon–1:00 P.M.	Campsite	Lunch	1 beer	Wife and sons	Lunch

Drinking Diary 3

Day of Week	Time of Drinking	Where	Occasion	Number and Type of Drinks	Number and Type of Companions	Foods—Snacks, etc.
Monday	None					
Tuesday	6:00 P.M.	Home	Dinner	1 glass wine	Husband drinking	Full meal
Wednesday	None					
Thursday	None					
Friday	None					
Saturday	8:00–10:30 P.M.	Restaurant	Dinner	1 Manhattan, 2 glasses wine	Husband and another couple	Full meal
Sunday	None					

136 / Personal Drinking Records

Drinking Diary 4

Day of Week	Time of Drinking	Where	Occasion	Number and Type of Drinks	Number and Type of Companions	Foods–Snacks, etc.
Monday	5:00–6:00 P.M.	Home	Before dinner	1 Manhattan	Alone	None
Monday	6:00–7:00 P.M.	Home	Before dinner	1 Manhattan	Husband drinking	None
Tuesday	5:00–6:00 P.M.	Home	Before dinner	1 Manhattan	Alone	None
Wednesday	5:30–6:00 P.M.	Home	Relaxing	1 martini	Alone	None
Wednesday	7:00–9:30 P.M.	Restaurant	Dinner	1 martini, ½ bottle wine, brandy Alexander	Husband and sons	Full meal
Thursday	5:00–6:00 P.M.	Home	Relaxing	1 whiskey sour	Alone	None
Friday	5:00–6:30 P.M.	Home	Before dinner	2 Manhattans	Alone	None
Friday	7:00–9:00 P.M.	Home	Dinner	1 Manhattan	Husband and sons	Full meal
Saturday	4:00–4:30 P.M.	Campsite	After hiking	1 beer	Husband and sons	Chips
Saturday	7:00–10:00 P.M.	Campsite	Relaxing	2 gin and tonics	Husband and sons	Snacks
Sunday	None					

Day of Week	Time of Drinking	Where	Occasion	Number and Type of Drinks	Number and Type of Companions	Foods—Snacks, etc.
Monday	10:30–11:30 P.M.	Restaurant-bar	Dinner	1 bottle beer	Alone	Full meal
Tuesday	None					
Wednesday	11:00–11:45 P.M.	Restaurant-bar	Dinner	2 glasses wine	Alone	Full meal
Thursday	10:30 P.M.–12:30 A.M.	Home	After date	2 gin and tonics	Boyfriend, who was drinking	Snacks
Friday	10:30–11:30 P.M.	Restaurant-bar	Dinner	2 glasses wine	Alone	Full meal
Saturday	4:30–5:30 P.M.	Home	Relaxing	1 gin and tonic	Roommate	None
Sunday	1:30–2:30 P.M.	Parents' home	Dinner	1 gin and tonic	Parents not drinking	Dinner

Drinking Diary 5

Day of Week	Time of Drinking	Where	Occasion	Number and Type of Drinks	Number and Type of Companions	Foods—Snacks, etc.
Monday	None					
Tuesday	None					
Wednesday	None					
Thursday	None					
Friday	None					
Saturday	7:30–11:00 P.M.	Friends' home	Visiting	2 gin and tonics	Husband and other couples	Snacks
Sunday	None					

Drinking Diary 6

PERSONAL DRINKING RECORDS

Day of Week	Time of Drinking	Where	Occasion	Number and Type of Drinks	Number and Type of Companions	Foods—Snacks, etc.
Monday	None					
Tuesday	None					
Wednesday	10:00–11:00 P.M.	Restaurant	After bowling	2 bottles beer	Wife and friends	Pizza
Thursday	None					
Friday	7:30–8:30 P.M.	Home	Supper	2 bottles beer	Wife not drinking	Full meal
Saturday	8:30–11:00 P.M.	Home	Friends visiting	1 bottle beer	Wife and another couple	Snacks
Sunday	4:00–5:00 P.M.	Neighbors' home	Visiting	1 bottle beer	Neighbors	None

Drinking Diary 7

Day of Week	Time of Drinking	Where	Occasion	Number and Type of Drinks	Number and Type of Companions	Foods—Snacks, etc.
Monday	5:00–7:00 P.M.	Bar	After work	4 glasses beer	2 male friends	Light meal
Tuesday	9:00–11:30 P.M.	Bar	Relaxing	6 bottles beer	Alone	None
Wednesday	7:00–10:00 P.M.	Friends' home	Visiting	2 bottles beer	Couple	None
Thursday	None					
Friday	5:00–8:00 P.M.	Bar	After work	6 bottles beer	1 male and 2 female friends	Snacks
Friday	8:00–9:30 P.M.	Restaurant	Supper	2 bottles beer	Same as above	Pizza
Friday	10:00 P.M.–1:00 A.M.	Bar	Relaxing	8 bottles beer	Same as above	Snacks
Saturday	4:00–5:00 P.M.	Home	Relaxing	1 bottle beer	Alone	None
Saturday	10:00 P.M.–1:00 A.M.	Bar	After movie	5 bottles beer	1 female	Snacks
Sunday	7:30–10:00 P.M.	Friends' home	Visiting	2 bottles beer	Another couple	None

Drinking Diary 8

Drinking Diary 9

Day of Week	Time of Drinking	Where	Occasion	Number and Type of Drinks	Number and Type of Companions	Foods—Snacks, etc.
Monday	None					
Tuesday	None					
Wednesday	10:00–11:00 P.M.	Restaurant	After bowling	1 bottle beer	Husband and friends	Pizza
Thursday	None					
Friday	None					
Saturday	None					
Sunday	None					

Drinking Diary 10

Day of Week	Time of Drinking	Where	Occasion	Number and Type of Drinks	Number and Type of Companions	Foods—Snacks, etc.
Monday	None					
Tuesday	None					
Wednesday	None					
Thursday	None					
Friday	6:00–7:00 P.M.	Home	Supper	1 bottle beer	Husband	Full meal
Saturday	None					
Sunday	None					

Drinking Diary 11

Day of Week	Time of Drinking	Where	Occasion	Number and Type of Drinks	Number and Type of Companions	Foods—Snacks, etc.
Monday	noon–12:30 P.M.	Tavern	Lunch	1 bottle beer	Alone	Sandwich
Tuesday	noon–12:30 P.M.	Tavern	Lunch	1 bottle beer	Alone	Sandwich
Wednesday	noon–12:30 P.M.	Tavern	Lunch	1 bottle beer	Alone	Sandwich
Wednesday	8:00–11:00 P.M.	Home	TV	2 bottles beer	Wife present, not drinking	Potato chips
Thursday	noon–12:30 P.M.	Tavern	Lunch	1 bottle beer	Alone	Sandwich
Friday	noon–12:30 P.M.	Tavern	Lunch	1 bottle beer	Alone	Sandwich
Saturday	2:30–4:00 P.M.	Home	TV	2 bottles beer	Alone	None
Sunday	None					

Day of Week	Time of Drinking	Where	Occasion	Number and Type of Drinks	Number and Type of Companions	Foods—Snacks, etc.
Monday	noon–1:00 P.M.	Home	Lunch	1 bottle beer	Alone	Sandwich
Monday	4:00–6:00 P.M.	Home	Supper	2 shots whiskey, 2 beers	Wife not drinking	Supper
Tuesday	noon–1:00 P.M.	Home	Lunch	1 beer	Alone	Sandwich
Tuesday	5:00–6:00 P.M.	Home	Supper	1 beer	Wife not drinking	Supper
Tuesday	8:00–11:00 P.M.	Home	TV	4 beers	Alone	None
Wednesday	noon–1:00 P.M.	Home	Lunch	1 beer	Alone	Sandwich
Wednesday	8:00–11:00 P.M.	Home	TV	2 beers	Wife not drinking	None
Thursday	noon–1:00 P.M.	Home	Lunch	1 beer	Alone	Sandwich
Thursday	3:00–5:00 P.M.	Home	Relaxing	2 shots whiskey, 2 beers	Alone	None
Thursday	7:30 P.M.–midnight	Home	TV	3 beers	Alone	None
Friday	noon–1:00 P.M.	Home	Lunch	1 beer	Alone	Sandwich
Saturday	2:00 A.M.	Home	After work	2 shots whiskey, 2 beers	Alone	Snacks
Saturday	noon–1:00 P.M.	Home	Lunch	1 beer	Alone	Sandwich
Sunday	2:00 A.M.	Home	After work	2 shots whiskey, 2 beers	Alone	Snacks
Sunday	noon–1:00 P.M.	Home	Lunch	1 beer	Alone	Sandwich
Sunday	4:00–5:00 P.M.	Home	TV	2 beers	Alone	None
Sunday	7:00–11:00 P.M.	Home	TV	3 beers	Wife not drinking	None

Drinking Diary 12

Drinking Diary 13

Day of Week	Time of Drinking	Where	Occasion	Number and Type of Drinks	Number and Type of Companions	Foods—Snacks, etc.
Infrequent Drinker—one or two glasses of wine on holidays.						

Drinking Diary 14

Day of Week	Time of Drinking	Where	Occasion	Number and Type of Drinks	Number and Type of Companions	Foods—Snacks, etc.
Infrequent drinking, once or twice a year.						

The sample diaries explained

There is no question that in the minds of most people alcohol use and misuse is a matter of personal choice and taste—or need, if you will. And it would seem to follow that drinking problems are born solely within the individual. But one matter continues to plague us, and that is the remarkably high incidence of alcohol problems in American, French, and Soviet societies (to note a few), as contrasted with others. Doesn't this mean we should examine the society instead of focusing entirely on the individual to determine the source of alcohol problems?

Looking only at heredity, physiology, or psychology certainly relieves us of any responsibility we, as a society, may feel about the serious plight of those with drinking problems. But how can we rationalize away the known differences in alcohol problems among nations?

As a psychiatrist, I would be the last to deny the importance of unconscious, uncontrollable pressures in the individual, but I am firmly convinced that the real force creating alcohol problems is sociocultural. And if, in fact, the demands of our society, life-style, and career shape our drinking patterns, then hopes for change are great.

A study of the situations in which drinking takes place may begin to reveal an essential determinant of alcohol use and misuse. It was as part of such a study that the drinking diaries were developed. Take a look at the diaries I have included and see how they illustrate the point.

These drinking diaries were filled in, for a typical week, by three couples and one single woman, for two different periods of time for each person. The first diary is that of a thirty-two-year-old man who is married and has two sons, aged six and four. Mr. Alon is a salesman of business machines who, at thirty-two, has the comfortable income of $26,000 per year and takes pride in his home and his college degree in business administration. He is a good person who enjoys his life, his wife, his sons, his work.

Notice how on Monday from 6:00 to 7:30 P.M., in the comfort

of his home, he takes two small martinis in that hour and a half, while his wife sips sherry. Mr. Alon does not eat anything during this time with his wife, but it does not require too vivid an imagination to see them sharing the day's events—he talking about his successful sales and near-sales, and some of the people he met that day, while she talks about the children and the concerns that her friends shared with her. It is a pleasant moment. Then, at 7:30 P.M., they go into the kitchen for dinner, and Mr. Alon sips two glasses of beer while his wife takes wine with the meal, and they continue their conversation. For both husband and wife, Monday is a beneficial drinking experience.

On Tuesday, the young man, while having his lunch in a restaurant from 11:30 to 1:30, drinks one martini before lunch and shares a bottle of wine with two colleagues.

But on Wednesday we see him in a different context: off on a business trip, sitting in a faraway place in a bar from 6:00 to 8:00 P.M., alone with chips and three martinis—much more than he had in the comfort of his home. And after his lonely cocktail hours, from 8:00 to 9:30 P.M., he consumes half a bottle of wine as solace for his loneliness at dinner. While still out of town on Thursday, at an extended luncheon with four business associates who all choose to drink, he consumes two martinis, two glasses of wine, and finishes one brandy after his meal. And that same Thursday, on the two-hour flight home, he has two martinis and a glass of wine.

If one wanted to focus on amount for the moment, we can see that when he leaves the comfort of his home territory and family and is in another context of drinking, Mr. Alon's consumption rises appreciably. On Friday, we see him at a buffet dinner party in a friend's home that goes on for some seven hours, during which he consumes two martinis, ten glasses of punch, and three bottles of beer.

Saturday finds him at his supper, accompanying his meal with two beers, and he anesthetizes a Sunday visit to his in-laws' home by accompanying his dinner with three gin and tonics.

In familiar and comfortable surroundings, the alcohol Mr.

Alon chooses to drink is gentle and beneficial, but a certain harshness creeps in when he is lonely or under stress.

In Drinking Diary 2, we again see Mr. Alon, who is now forty-five and a business executive in a large corporation with an income of some $42,000 per year. Mr. Alon's sons are now nineteen and seventeen years of age. And we see that on this Monday one martini suffices for the former two and beer does not accompany the dinner. The Tuesday business lunch is not appreciably different from the one thirteen years before, but his general shift is to some leisurely drinking and sharing with his wife and sons, and only seems to heighten in business or social situations.

The older Mr. Alon needs alcohol less and is more relaxed about his drinking but nevertheless reflects the contexts in which he takes his alcohol. In his younger years not a day went by without some alcohol, but we note in this diary that he drank none at all on Thursday.

Now look at the Drinking Diary (3) of his wife Alice. In the first diary, Alice is thirty, a graduate of secretarial school, and now a housewife. It does not take much looking at her diary to see that her drinking during one week includes only a glass of wine on Tuesday at dinner with her husband, and one Manhattan and two glasses of wine when they are at a restaurant on Saturday.

But then we see Alice some thirteen years later (Diary 4). Certainly her children, at nineteen and seventeen, are no longer very dependent on her. And her husband, now enjoying his success and feeling less uncertain about his work, probably has fewer problems to share with Alice. We see that she has one Manhattan alone before her husband comes home, shares another with him before dinner, and seems to have shifted her drinking patterns to center around her aloneness. Alcohol is now more important in her life and less important to her husband. As their situations have changed, so has their drinking.

Neither amounts nor the time or reason for drinking indicates that either of these people has a problem. But I have little doubt that if Alice's emotional needs and isolation are not attended to, there's great potential for serious problems.

The next diary we will examine (Drinking Diary 5) belongs to Sharon, aged twenty-four and single, who is a part-time waitress in a bar and a part-time college student. Sharon is proud of having completed three years of college as an English major. She shares a lovely apartment with one roommate. We can see that late in the evening, when she has finished her classes and waiting on people, Sharon takes a beer with her dinner. On Tuesday, when she devotes all of her energies to her college work and does not work in the restaurant-bar, she has no alcohol at all. But Wednesday finds her back at work, and so two glasses of wine go along with dinner. And on Thursday, at home after a date, she joins her boyfriend, who is drinking, taking two gin and tonics over the course of two hours. On Friday, work at the restaurant-bar has her enjoying some wine with a meal. On Saturday, she has a gin and tonic with her roommate, as she does at Sunday dinner at her parents' home.

Then we see Sharon eleven years later (Diary 6), married to a prospering dentist and with two children aged three and one and a half. Her diary is rather empty except for Saturday night, when she takes two gin and tonics in the course of the evening, visiting at the home of friends with her husband and other couples. Sharon's career and situation have changed and so has her use of alcohol.

And then there is Billy (Diary 7), aged twenty-seven, married, without children, who is a typesetter with an annual income of $12,000. Billy rents an apartment and is a high school graduate with one year's experience as a part-time college student. Billy takes some beer with pizza at a restaurant after bowling with his wife and friends, or at supper, or in other social situations, but outside these contexts he does not drink at all on three days.

Eight years later, Billy, at age thirty-five (Diary 8), is now divorced, and although he continues to make beer his only alcoholic drink, his pattern of drinking has changed. Without a wife to share his life, he takes beer either with friends in a bar or alone in bars. Most of his drinking is done outside the home, either alone or with friends or with women companions. The relationship of his drinking to food is minimal. The change in his life and its impact on his drinking is plain to see.

His former wife, Susan (Diary 9), illustrates an interesting comparison. She is twenty-four years old, working as a secretary, and adding her $7,500 annual income to their mutual resources. Her drinking diary during this period is blank, except for one bottle of beer that she had while with her husband and friends after bowling.

Eight years later (Diary 10), Susan, now thirty-two, after her divorce from Billy, is remarried to a factory foreman and has one child, aged four. And her drinking diary remains the same—essentially blank, except for that one beer taken at supper at home with her husband. Susan's context and career have not essentially changed and neither has her drinking pattern.

Edward (Diary 11), a fifty-two-year-old man who is married and has no children, earns an income of $16,000 per year as a factory worker on an auto assembly line and owns his own home. He has a high school education. He takes a beer with his lunch or while watching TV alone at home or in a tavern.

But Edward now (Diary 12) can be seen in his new role at age sixty-three, retired, earning $10,000 per year in his part-time work as night watchman. His active life and feelings of self-worth have changed, and instead of drinking mainly in taverns, he drinks at home and with greater frequency. He has added harder liquor, the amounts are greater, and although essentially he still drinks alone, where and how he is using alcohol show a shift that has ominous implications.

Edward's wife Molly (Diaries 13 and 14), is a high school graduate. She is a housewife, childless, and active in her church. At fifty she's an infrequent drinker, taking an occasional glass of wine on holidays. Eleven years later she has essentially the same life and maintains her old drinking pattern.

With a comparison of these diaries we begin to perceive a new way of looking at an old problem. At no time in their histories do we talk about these people as being drunk or dysfunctional. They have not lost work because of their drinking, they have not been arrested, and they have not illustrated most of the stereotypical drinking problems. Yet, in two individuals a change in the context and career prompts a change in the drinking pattern that is potentially serious. These diaries are not dramatic examples of how societies cause people to focus more or less on alcohol and its use, but they are intriguing clues that cry out for further investigation by serious students of alcohol use and abuse.

Steps and Actions

Here for quick review and easy reference are the fundamental steps and actions that will help you get the most from drinking.

Step 1: Food

1. Provide food for yourself or your guests before drinking.

2. Serve bulky food such as Italian or French bread, cheese, meats, and creamy spreads (see list on page 186).

3. Avoid such food as pretzels, potato chips, and salty snacks. They lack bulk and increase thirst. Taking a lot of alcohol to quench an unquenchable thirst is not the best way to go.

4. Vegetables or crackers are inadequate alone. Serve them only if you are serving bulkier foods as well.

5. Wait fifteen minutes after eating before sipping alcohol.

Most important: food before drink.
Next in importance: food with drink.
Least important: food after drink.

Step 2: Paraphernalia

1. Measure the alcohol in a drink. A one-ounce jigger is the right size.

2. For mixed drinks, use a tall, small-diameter glass.

3. For beer, use no larger than an eight-ounce glass.

4. For wine, use no larger than a six-ounce glass, filled no more than halfway.

5. Never pour alcohol unmeasured from a bottle.

Remember: You are dispensing a drug.
The only drug whose dose is unmeasured is alcohol, except in bars where it is measured for economic, not safety, purposes.

Step 3: Dilution

1. Always fill a glass above the brim with ice cubes. We want as much ice in the glass as we can get before the drink is poured, since alcohol makes the ice settle.

2. Use only small-sized ice cubes. Large ice cubes leave big spaces to be filled with alcohol. Small ice cubes in a proper glass make a one-ounce drink appear ample.

3. Have ice cubes readily available and in everyone's sight. People tend to add cubes automatically to their drinks as the level diminishes.

4. Use water as a mixer. It is the best diluter of alcohol.

5. Avoid carbonated mixers.

Remember: The appearance and size of a drink satisfies a person as much as the alcoholic content—unless he is out to get bombed!

Step 4: Sound

1. Choose a quiet place. Soft, gentle music or low levels of noise are the best background for drinking. Soft sounds diminish tensions—less alcohol is required for relaxation, and the reaction to the amount consumed is pleasanter.

2. Avoid loud music or other noise. Loud, harsh sounds increase isolation. We therefore talk louder and become charged up, trying to overcome the din. More alcohol is needed to feel relaxed, and the reaction to alcohol is likely to be increased aggressiveness.

Step 5: Hosting

1. Have a fixed drinking period of not more than one hour before dinner. Serve each guest no more than two one-ounce

glasses of distilled spirits measured by a jigger and preferably diluted; no more than three eight-ounce glasses of beer; or no more than two half glasses of wine.

2. When wine accompanies a meal, serve no more than two half-filled glasses of wine per person.

3. If cocktails or wine have been served earlier, brandy or after-dinner drinks should be served only when the period of dining has taken more than a minimum of one and one-half hours.

4. Try not to offer or serve any alcohol later than forty-five minutes before the guests are expected to leave.

5. Create a drinking atmosphere conducive to healthy, safe, and careful drinking by providing lots of light and a circular seating arrangement. Studies have shown that fluorescent lights, especially pink ones, create tension and irritability, so it's just as well to avoid them. What we want is pleasant, soft light that makes everyone in the group comfortably visible.

6. What we reflect and expect is what we'll get from our guests. We don't want to make them sick with our food; we don't want to make them sick with our drinks.

Step 6: Bars and Cocktail Lounges

1. Select a well-lighted bar. Dim and dark surroundings suggest mystery and intrigue or isolation, which can cause mild, barely noticed, tenseness. Tenseness creates a tendency to overdrink.

2. Select a place where seating arrangements allow people to notice and be aware of each other. In general, booths are bad—they increase our isolation and separateness and push us toward heavier drinking. Of course, with this, as with every rule, there are exceptions. A quiet drink with someone special in a comfortable booth can be a beneficial drinking experience. Bars should be circular, not linear. Facing people across a well-lighted

circular bar is conducive to moderate drinking. Facing a wall, and not people, increases isolation and drinking.

Step 7: Preparation

1. One person should take the responsibility of preparing and serving the drinks. Each guest should *not* pour his own drink. You are really dispensing a drug, and you should control the dosage—if you want your guests to enjoy all the advantages of drinking. Besides, it's just plain good manners to serve your guests.

2. The alcohol supply should always be in a separate room. Guests who are not made to feel free to serve themselves will delay before asking someone else to get another. Also, alcohol out of sight is alcohol not so much in mind. A study of overeaters reveals that if an extra supply of food is around but out of their sight, they eat average amounts. When they can see it, they gorge. Supermarkets understand this impulse—they create lavish displays of their products so we'll buy more.

Step 8: Ways of Offering a Drink

Kindness	**Cornering**
1. Would you like *something* to drink?	1. How about a drink?
2. What do you want to drink?	2. You want a drink, don't you?
3. Can I get you a drink?	3. You look like you need a drink.
	4. Do you want a drink?
	5. Come on, have a drink.

Action 1: When a guest is gulping drinks

1. Freshen the drink only with ice cubes, actively offering to add ice to the drink.

2. Delay getting the second drink.

3. Actively push food on the guest.

4. Cut the dose of the next drink in half.

Action 2: When we're on the "martini circuit" but don't want to drink

Order:
1. A Virgin Mary
2. Club soda and orange juice
3. Perrier water
4. 7-Up and grenadine
5. Bitter Lemon straight
6. Iced tea
7. Lemonade
8. Tonic water and lime
9. Piña colada without rum

Neither drinkers nor nondrinkers will be uptight if you are holding a glass containing a beverage that looks alcoholic. The above drinks—and others—allow people the illusion that we are drinking with them.

Action 3: When someone is pushing drinks on us

1. Ask for the drink "neat" in a jigger with the mix in a side glass. We control our own dose and alcohol concentration this way.

2. Always keep the glass topped off—by adding ice.

3. Tell them you are hungry, not thirsty—spend time with food.

4. Say "No, thank you!" firmly, but with a smile.

Action 4: When someone at home is drinking too much and doesn't believe it

1. Get them to mark the bottle of their favorite drink with a felt pen or Scotch Tape. Keep them marking the level and attaching the tape strips to provide visual evidence of the diminishing fluid level.

2. Ask them if you may take a Polaroid picture of them after they've had a lot to drink. (Get permission in writing.)

3. Ask them if you may make a tape recording of how they sound with a lot of liquor in their system.

Note: No one but the drinker himself gets to see the bottle or picture or hear the record. They're for the eyes and ears of the disbelieving drinker only. Seeing the level drop precipitously is believing. A picture or recording may be unkind, but letting someone drown in heavy drinking is cruel.

Action 5: In restaurants and bars

1. Don't let the waiter push or rush drinks.

2. Follow Anstie's limit.

3. Drink only when you really want it.

4. Keep the cork of the bottle handy—you may want to restopper unused wine (too often we drink more than we want for fear of wasting).

Action 6: If you've had a drunken party

1. Examine and discuss what in the atmosphere you created led to overdrinking.

2. Did you serve heavily dosed drinks to avoid the accusation of being stingy?

3. Did you highlight the capacity of people to drink; for example, "Boy, he can really hold his booze!"?

4. Are you really telling your guests that they can stand one another only when anesthetized?

Action 7: If you drink and have children

1. Explain to your children what you know about alcohol.

2. Ask them to tell you what they think about, and know of, drinking.

3. Let them have a taste of your drink if they ask.

4. Teach them—by example—how to drink responsibly.

Action 8: If you don't drink and have children

1. Explain to your children what you know about alcohol.

2. Tell them why you choose not to drink.

3. Tell them *your* preference about whether or not they decide to drink.

4. Let them know that they can tell you if they decide to drink.

5. Teach them the steps and actions of responsible drinking—even if they choose not to drink.

6. Don't create the lure of the forbidden by making too much of a fuss about alcohol.

Action 9: When you want to refuse a drink

1. Say "No, thank you." Suggest the substitute you'd prefer.

Remember: A "No" that is meant is usually accepted.

Action 10: Talking to a friend who drinks too much

1. Try to examine your own feelings first.

2. Ask yourself whether you are *truly* concerned, or just enjoying feeling superior.

3. If you're satisfied with your feelings and answers, then say whatever you feel.

The sound and feeling of concern are more important than the words you choose to use. Preaching, anger, aggressiveness, righteousness drive drinking-problem people to drink more.

Action 11: Helping a spouse to recognize that she (or he) has a problem and talk about it openly

1. Ask her to fill in a drinking diary (see page 131).

2. Compare the daily amounts consumed against Anstie's limits.

3. Mutually agree, in writing, to set a limit to the amount and frequency of drinking. If one drop more is used, or a period of drinking beyond that agreed to occurs, the spouse will agree there's a problem and discuss it. If the goal is achieved, the other spouse will shut up about it.

4. Set a period of abstinence from alcohol.

If achieved: no discussion.
If failed: we talk.

Action 12: Handling people who insist that you drink with them

1. Show them a nonalcoholic look-alike drink (see page 158).

2. Tell them you can't stand the taste.

3. Tell them alcohol makes you ill.

4. As a last resort, ask them: (a) Why is it important to them to make you drink when you choose not to? (b) What hang-up do they have about booze?

We need never be defensive if we choose not to drink. The people who push us to drink ought to be defensive.

Action 13: When you must deal with an employee whose drinking interferes with his (or her) work

1. Find out what treatment programs exist in your community.

2. Explore the location of occupational alcoholism programs in your area.

3. Take the employee out to a lunch without drinks and gently tell him the problem as you see it.

4. Offer every assistance in getting him to a treatment program.

5. Give him a little time (a few weeks) to come to terms with the idea.

6. If he refuses, tell him he will need to look elsewhere for employment.

A caring employer aids the healthy functioning of his employees, treating all illnesses alike. If an employee continues to be too ill to function, a replacement becomes necessary.

Action 14: When you want to help a friend who is alcoholic

1. Explore the treatment facilities in your community.

2. Speak to affiliates of the National Council on Alcoholism in your community about a referral.

3. Find out about local AA meetings.

4. Offer to go with your friend to any treatment resource he or she chooses for as long as he or she wishes.

Support, caring, and concern (shown instead of stated) are the best help.

Action 15: When a companion is drunk

1. Let him sleep, if possible.

2. Do not let him drive.

3. Drive him home, or call a cab to take him home.

4. Encourage him to stay where he is overnight.

5. Take a long walk with him to provide time for oxidation to take place.

6. If all else fails, call the cops; better an angry friend than a dead one.

Appendix I
Effects of Specific Medication When Combined with Alcohol *

Narcotic agents such as **Dilaudid** or **Demerol** or **Darvon** are themselves depressant agents of the central nervous system and are potentiated by alcohol. The combination can cause enough depression of the center that controls breathing to stop the breathing completely.

Combining some antibiotics like the sulfanamids and chloromycetin with alcohol causes flushing, headache, nausea, and vomiting. But this is very rare and not the severe kind of difficulty that can result from other combinations.

For some unexplained reason, alcohol seems to speed up the normal rate of metabolizing the anticonvulsant drug **Dilantin,** so that its useful effects disappear sooner than usual. An epileptic person who is under treatment with **Dilantin,** and free of seizures, may have a seizure after prolonged heavy drinking.

Antihistamines are sedative in effect, and in combination with alcohol they become strongly so. It is hazardous to drive or perform any complicated tasks while taking alcohol and anti-

---

* A major resource for the information in this section was a paper entitled "Drug Interactions with Alcohol," by James Coleman and William E. Evans, which appeared in the winter 1975–76 edition of *Alcohol Health and Research World.*

histamines. There is just no question that the person who wants to be safe should never take alcohol when on antihistamine medication.

Now, if you're on an antihypertensive drug, there is no evidence that alcohol will produce any unhealthy effects. As a matter of fact, some people believe that combining alcohol with **Reserpine** or **Aldomet, Apresoline** or **Dralzine,** or **Esimil, Ismelin** (or any of the diuretic drugs used to control high blood pressure) increases the drug's effectiveness.

Disulfiram **(Antabuse)** is used to enforce abstinence from drinking. When combined with alcohol it can produce a very unpleasant feeling of flushing, a painful throbbing in the head and neck, headaches, difficulty in breathing, nausea and vomiting, and almost any other uncomfortable symptom you can imagine. Some people who are being treated with this drug to control problem drinking may be tempted to take a chance and have a drink anyway. I strongly advise against taking alcohol if there is any possibility that even a small level of disulfiram remains in the blood.

There appears to be no problem in taking alcohol with diuretic medication. Some people contend that retaining water may be one of the major problems of chronic heavy drinkers, and since diuretics help eliminate water, they may even be helpful.

In dealing with drugs that lower the blood sugar (used in treating hyperglycemia), we have to remember that alcohol also tends, in some people, to lower the blood sugar level. In these cases, taking alcohol will further lower the blood sugar level. This problem is more common in thin people.

Oral insulin **(Diabinese; Orinase),** which is a hypoglycemic drug used to lower blood sugar, may produce an Antabuse-like reaction if you take alcohol with it. And this medication tends to metabolize faster following the intake of large amounts of alcohol. I would warn that the response to alcohol's interaction with hypoglycemic agents is unpredictable and potentially severe, so it is best to take no alcohol, or use it with extreme caution.

The major tranquilizers and antidepressant drugs, the phenothiazines—for example, **Tindal** or **Repoise, Thorazine, Prolixin, Mellaril,** and **Compazine**—are among a large class of drugs widely used to treat psychotic patients. In combination with alcohol, they produce an additive central nervous system effect that results in depression of the respiratory control centers. The other danger is that the phenothiazines are metabolized in the liver, and this may cause some complications in heavy drinkers who have liver problems.

Our brains have automatic controls that prevent convulsions (the level of control is called the seizure threshold). Certain conditions—high fever, for instance—may lower the seizure threshold level. Phenothiazines can also lower the seizure threshold, and when they're combined with heavy drinking there is a greater general risk of convulsion. Phenothiazines tend to cause some irregular heart rhythms, and alcohol can intensify them once they begin. These drugs also lead to lower blood pressure.

Such common antidepressant drugs as **Elavil, Norpramin, Tofrānil, Aventyl,** and **Sinequan** reinforce the depressing effects of alcohol on the central nervous system. There are reports of people who have been killed while trying to operate machinery or drive while under the influence of these combinations. These drugs are also capable of lowering the seizure threshold and aggravating epilepsy. One must be particularly careful when combining alcohol with antidepressant medications if there is evidence of liver difficulty.

Other types of antidepressant drugs (the monoamine-oxidase inhibitors), such as **Marplan, Eutonyl,** and **Nardil,** are better not used with alcohol because they tend to slow the metabolism of alcohol and strengthen the central nervous system depressant effect. There is sometimes even an Antabuse type of reaction. Some people get a sudden rapid rise in blood pressure when they are using this class of antidepressant drugs and take certain alcoholic drinks, such as Chianti wine and beer. So it is better that they not use alcohol when they are on this medication.

The largest group of widely used drugs, collectively known as sedative-hypnotics, includes barbiturates and minor tranquilizers. Their action is very similar to that of alcohol and, as you would guess, the combination of any of these drugs with alcohol will result in an increased, bizarre effect on the central nervous system with a decrease of alertness and judgment, impairment of motor coordination and manual skills, and, in some drugs, a dangerously severe lowering of the blood pressure. Some of these drugs, **Valium,** for instance, may very well affect a person's tolerance for alcohol. The combination can affect heart functioning and cause circulatory and respiratory collapse.

Chloral hydrate is another drug that creates a depressant effect with alcohol. This is a drug used in a "Mickey Finn," a drink that has been known to cause respiratory arrest and death. Chloral hydrate should not be used with alcohol.

Such stimulants as amphetamine and caffeine, when taken with alcohol, make us appear more alert but do not really relieve the depressant effect of the alcohol or improve functioning. As a matter of fact, they can produce bizarre effects on the cardiovascular system, including some hypertension (high blood pressure) and rapid heartbeat, and could be very serious in people already having difficulties with their circulatory system. Combined with alcohol, they can produce convulsive disorders.

Many things affect a patient's response to medication, including the functioning of his kidneys or liver and his allergic responses, but it is important to keep in mind that alcohol is frequently overlooked as a possible complicator. A list of these common drugs and their possible effects in combination with alcohol can be found in Appendix II.

Appendix II
Alcohol and Drugs ⁕

Drugs with Alcohol   **Possible Effects**

1. Analgesics
   Narcotic (morphine, codeine, meperidine [Demerol], methadone) — Respiratory arrest. Unpredictable depression of brain activity.
   Nonnarcotic (salicylates—aspirin) — Stomach irritation. Increased gastric bleeding.

2. Anesthetics (general)
   With alcohol — Additive depressant effect.
   Without alcohol — High doses required for effect in alcoholics.

3. Antialcohol (Antabuse, calcium carbamide) — Nausea, vomiting, headache, blood pressure rise, heart irregular, occasional death.

4. Antidiabetic (insulin, oral medication) — Hypoglycemia, severe (exaggerated insulin response).

5. Antihistamines (hay-fever medication, Benadryl, Coricidin, Contac, and so on) — Increased sedative action.

⁕ Adapted from information furnished by the National Clearing House for Alcohol Information.

Drugs with Alcohol	Possible Effects
6. Antihypertensives (reserpine, deserpidine, guanethidine, mecalymine, and so on)	Increase of hypotension. Increase of sedation.
7. Anticoagulants (acenocoumarol, phenindamine, and so on)	Decreased anticoagulant effect.
8. Anticonvulsant (Dilantin)	Decreased anticonvulsant effect.
9. Antidepressants (imipramine, doxepin, monoamine-oxidase inhibitors, and so on)	Increased sedation (Chianti wine especially to be avoided).
10. Central nervous system stimulants (amphetamine, caffeine, and so on)	False sense of security.
11. Diuretics (thiazide, quinethazone, furosemide, and so on)	Hypotension.
12. Sedative-hypnotics (barbiturates, nonbarbiturates, bromides, and so on)	Severe sedation, coma, respiratory arrest, death.

13. Tranquilizers
  Minor (diazepam, meprobamate)
  Major (phenothiazines, and so on)
	Severe sedation.
	Impaired motor skills.

14. Vitamins (B12, B1, folic acid, Vitamins A, D, E, K)	Decreased absorption with heavy drinking.

Appendix III
Alcohol Content *

Beer: varies from 2 to 8 percent.
    2 percent in mild Scandinavian beer and Russian kvass.
    3.2 percent in some military and college campus beers.
    4.5 percent in most American beers.
    8 percent in especially strong beers.

Dry wines (natural and unfortified): 8 to 12 percent.
    For example, Burgundy, Chianti, sauterne.
    Most U.S. table wines are 12 to 14 percent.

Vermouth-aperitif wines: 18 percent.

Dessert, sweet, cocktail wines: 20 percent.
    For example, sherry, port, muscatel.

Spirits: 40 to 50 percent.
    For example, vodka, rum, whiskey, gin, brandy, liqueurs.

Cordials: 25 to 40 percent.
    For example, blackberry, maraschino, curaçao, anisette.

Note: Percentages are by volume—the proportion of alcohol in the fluid volume. Since fermentation goes no higher than 14 percent, fortified wines have alcohol or brandy added to them, while distillation brings the alcohol content of the others up. Low-percentage drinks are the result of drawing off the product early.

* Based on information from an article entitled "Alcohol Consumption," by Mark Keller, which appeared in *Encylopaedia Britannica*, 15th ed., 1974, p. 437.

Appendix IV

Blood Alcohol Concentrations *

(Approximations for Statistical Populations Only)

Concentration

0.05 percent (1 part alcohol to 2,000 parts blood)
3 ounces distilled spirits in 2 hours

0.08 percent (1 part alcohol to 1,500 parts blood)
4½ ounces distilled spirits in 2 hours

0.10 percent (1 part alcohol to 1,000 parts blood)
6 ounces distilled spirits in 2 hours

0.20 percent (1 part alcohol to 500 parts blood)
10 ounces distilled spirits in 2 hours

Effect

Loosening of judgment, thought, and restraint.
Release of tension; carefree sensation.

Tensions and inhibitions of everyday life lessened.

Voluntary motor action affected: hand and arm movements, walk, and speech clumsy.

Severe impairment: staggering, loud, incoherent, emotionally unstable, very drunk.
100 times greater traffic accident risk.

* Adapted from information furnished by the National Clearing House for Alcohol Information.

Concentration	Effect
0.30 percent (1 part alcohol to 300 parts blood) 14 ounces distilled spirits in 2 hours	Deeper areas of brain affected. Parts affecting stimulus response and understanding confused, stuporous.
0.40 percent (1 part alcohol to 250 parts blood) 18 ounces distilled spirits in 2 hours	Asleep, difficult to arouse, incapable of voluntary action, surgical anesthesia.
0.50 percent (1 part alcohol to 200 parts blood) 22 ounces distilled spirits in 2 hours	Coma, anesthesia of centers controlling breathing and heartbeat. Death.

Appendix V*

State Alcoholism Authorities and Program Contacts

Officially Designated Authority   **Program Contact**

Alabama

Department of Mental Health
502 Washington Avenue
Montgomery, Alabama 36104

Alabama State Alcoholism Program
145 Moulton Street
Montgomery, Alabama 36104
Telephone: (205) 265-2301 X-235

Alaska

Department of Health and Social
    Services
Pouch H
Juneau, Alaska 99801

Division of Family and Children's
    Services
Office of Alcoholism
Pouch HO5F
Juneau, Alaska 99801
Telephone: (907) 586-6201

Arizona

Department of Health Services
State Health Building
1740 West Adams Street
Phoenix, Arizona 85007

Community Programs
2500 East Van Buren Street
Phoenix, Arizona 85008
Telephone: (602) 271-3438

* Adapted from information furnished by the National Clearing House for Alcohol Information.

Officially Designated Authority *Program Contact*

Arkansas

Department of Social and Rehabilitative Services
406 National Old Line Building
Little Rock, Arkansas 72201

Office of Alcohol Abuse and Alcoholism
1515 West Seventh Street, Suite 202
Little Rock, Arkansas 72202
Telephone: (501) 371-2003

California

Office of Alcoholism
825 Fifteenth Street
Sacramento, California 95814

Office of Alcoholism
825 Fifteenth Street
Sacramento, California 95814
Telephone: (916) 445-1940

Colorado

Department of Health
Executive Director
4210 East Eleventh Avenue
Denver, Colorado 80220

Alcohol and Drug Abuse Division
4210 East Eleventh Avenue
Denver, Colorado 80220
Telephone: (303) 388-6111

Connecticut

Connecticut State Alcohol Council (Commissioner, Department of Mental Health)
90 Washington Street
Hartford, Connecticut 06115

Connecticut State Alcohol Council
90 Washington Street
Hartford, Connecticut 06115
Telephone: (203) 566-3464

Delaware

Department of Health and Social Services
Delaware State Hospital
New Castle, Delaware 19720

Alcoholism Services
3000 Newport Gap Pike
Wilmington, Delaware 19808
Telephone: (302) 998-0483

District of Columbia

Department of Human Resources
District Building
Washington, D.C. 20004

Department of Human Resources
District Building
Washington, D.C. 20004
Telephone: (202) 629-5443

Officially Designated Authority   *Program Contact*

Florida

Department of Health and Rehabilitative Services
1323 Winewood Boulevard
Tallahassee, Florida 32301

Mental Health Program Office
Alcoholic Rehabilitation Program
1309 Winewood Boulevard
Room 336
Tallahassee, Florida 32301
Telephone: (904) 488-6915

Guam

Guam Memorial Hospital
Agana, Guam 96910

Guam Memorial Hospital
Agana, Guam 96910

Georgia

Department of Human Resources
Commissioner
47 Trinity Avenue, S.W.
Atlanta, Georgia 30334

Division of Mental Health
Alcohol and Drug Abuse Services Section
618 Ponce de Leon Avenue, N.E.
Atlanta, Georgia 30308
Telephone: (404) 894-4785

Hawaii

Department of Health
1250 Punchbowl Street
Honolulu, Hawaii 96813

Substance Abuse Agency
1270 Queen Emma Street
Room 404
Honolulu, Hawaii 96813
Telephone: (808) 548-7655

Idaho

Department of Health and Welfare
Statehouse
Boise, Idaho 83720

Bureau of Substance Abuse
Statehouse, LBJ Building
Boise, Idaho 83720
Telephone: (208) 384-3920

Officially Designated Authority *Program Contact*

Illinois

Department of Mental Health and Developmental Disabilities
160 North LaSalle Street
Chicago, Illinois 60601

Department of Mental Health and Developmental Disabilities
Alcoholism Division
188 West Randolph Street
Room 1900
Chicago, Illinois 60601
Telephone: (312) 793-2907

Indiana

Department of Mental Health
1315 West Tenth Street
Indianapolis, Indiana 46202

Division of Addiction Services
Five Indiana Square
Indianapolis, Indiana 46204
Telephone: (317) 633-4477

Iowa

Division of Alcoholism
Lucas State Office Building
Des Moines, Iowa 50319

Division of Alcoholism
Lucas State Office Building
Des Moines, Iowa 50319
Telephone: (515) 281-5604

Kansas

Department of Social and Rehabilitation Services
Sixth Floor State Office Building
Topeka, Kansas 66612

Alcohol and Drug Abuse Section
535 Kansas Avenue
Room 1106
Topeka, Kansas 66603
Telephone: (913) 296-3991

Kentucky

Department of Human Resources
Capitol Annex
Frankfort, Kentucky 40601

Bureau of Health Services
275 East Main Street
Frankfort, Kentucky 40601
Telephone: (502) 564-3970

Officially Designated Authority	Program Contact

Louisiana

Division of Hospitals
200 Lafayette Street
Seventh Floor
Weber Building
Baton Rouge, Louisiana 70801

Bureau of Substance Abuse
200 Lafayette Street
Seventh Floor
Weber Building
Baton Rouge, Louisiana 70801
Telephone: (504) 389-2534

Maine

Department of Health and Welfare
Statehouse
Augusta, Maine 04330

Bureau of Rehabilitation
Office of Alcoholism and Drug Abuse
  Prevention
32 Winthrop Street
Augusta, Maine 04330
Telephone: (207) 289-2141

Maryland

Department of Health and Mental
  Hygiene
201 West Preston Street
Baltimore, Maryland 21201

Division of Alcoholism Control
201 West Preston Street
Baltimore, Maryland 21201
Telephone: (301) 383-2782

Massachusetts

Department of Public Health
600 Washington Street
Room 214
Boston, Massachusetts 02111

Division of Alcoholism
755 Boylston Street
Boston, Massachusetts 02116
Telephone: (617) 536-6983

Michigan

Department of Public Health
3500 North Logan Street
Lansing, Michigan 48914

Office of Substance Abuse Services
3500 North Logan Street
Lansing, Michigan 48914
Telephone: (517) 373-8600

Officially Designated Authority   *Program Contact*

Minnesota

Chemical Dependency Program Division
Metro Square Building
Room 402
Saint Paul, Minnesota 55101

Chemical Dependency Program Division
Metro Square Building
Room 402
Saint Paul, Minnesota 55101
Telephone: (612) 296-4610

Mississippi

Department of Mental Health
607 Robert E. Lee Office Building
Jackson, Mississippi 39201

Division of Alcohol Abuse and Alcoholism
125 Lelia Court
Jackson, Mississippi 39216
Telephone: (601) 354-7031

Missouri

Department of Mental Health
722 Jefferson Street
Jefferson City, Missouri 65101

Division of Alcoholism and Drug Abuse
P.O. Box 687
2002 Missouri Boulevard
Jefferson City, Missouri 65101
Telephone: (314) 751-4122

Montana

Department of Institutions
1539 Eleventh Avenue
Helena, Montana 59601

Division of Addictive Diseases
1539 Eleventh Avenue
Helena, Montana 59601
Telephone: (406) 449-3965

Nebraska

Division of Alcoholism
Box 94728
Lincoln, Nebraska 68509

Division of Alcoholism
Box 94728
Lincoln, Nebraska 68509
Telephone: (402) 471-2851

Officially Designated Authority   *Program Contact*

Nevada

Department of Human Resources
308 North Curry Street
Carson City, Nevada 89701

Bureau of Alcohol and Drug Abuse
Capitol Complex
1803 North Carson Street
Carson City, Nevada 89701
Telephone: (702) 885-4790

New Hampshire

Governor
Statehouse
Concord, New Hampshire 03301

Program of Alcohol and Drug Abuse
61 South Spring Street
Concord, New Hampshire 03301
Telephone: (603) 271-3531

New Jersey

State Department of Health
P.O. Box 1540
John Fitch Plaza
Trenton, New Jersey 08625

Alcohol, Narcotics, and Drug Abuse Unit
Alcoholism Control Program
P.O. Box 1540
John Fitch Plaza
Trenton, New Jersey 08625
Telephone: (609) 292-8947

New Mexico

Department of Hospitals and Institutions
425 Old Santa Fe Trail
Santa Fe, New Mexico 87501

New Mexico Commission on Alcoholism
P.O. Box 1731
Albuquerque, New Mexico 87103
Telephone: (505) 827-3251

New York

Department of Mental Hygiene
44 Holland Avenue
Albany, New York 12208

Division of Alcoholism
44 Holland Avenue
Albany, New York 12208
Telephone: (518) 474-5417

Officially Designated Authority *Program Contact*

North Carolina

Department of Human Resources
P.O. Box 26327
Raleigh, North Carolina 27611

Division of Mental Health Services
Alcohol and Drug Services
P.O. Box 26327
Raleigh, North Carolina 27611
Telephone: (919) 829-4670

North Dakota

State Department of Health
State Capitol
Bismarck, North Dakota 58501

Division of Alcoholism and Drug Abuse
909 Basin Avenue
Bismarck, North Dakota 58505
Telephone: (701) 224-2767

Ohio

Ohio Department of Health
450 East Town Street
P.O. Box 118
Columbus, Ohio 43216

Alcoholism Unit
450 East Town Street
P.O. Box 118
Columbus, Ohio 43216
Telephone: (614) 466-3445

Oklahoma

Department of Mental Health
408-A North Walnut Street
Oklahoma City, Oklahoma 73105

Division of Alcoholism
408-A North Walnut Street
Oklahoma City, Oklahoma 73105
Telephone: (405) 521-2811

Oregon

Department of Human Resources
318 Public Services Building
Salem, Oregon 97310

Mental Health Division
Programs for Alcohol and Drug Abuse
2570 Center Street, N.E.
Salem, Oregon 97310
Telephone: (503) 378-2163

Officially Designated Authority   *Program Contact*

Pennsylvania

Governor's Council on Drug and Alcohol Abuse
Office of the Governor
Commonwealth of Pennsylvania
2101 North Front Street
Harrisburg, Pennsylvania 17110

Governor's Council on Drug and Alcohol Abuse
Office of the Governor
Commonwealth of Pennsylvania
2101 North Front Street
Harrisburg, Pennsylvania 17110
Telephone: (717) 787-9857

Puerto Rico

Department of Addiction Services
Box B-Y
Rio Piedras, Puerto Rico 00928

State Alcoholism Program
Assistant Secretary for Alcoholism
Box B-Y
Rio Piedras, Puerto Rico 00928
Telephone: (809) 763-7575

Rhode Island

Department of Mental Health, Retardation and Hospitals
The Aime J. Forand Building
600 New London Avenue
Cranston, Rhode Island 02920

Services for Alcoholics
The Aime J. Forand Building
600 New London Avenue
Cranston, Rhode Island 02920
Telephone: (401) 464-3291

American Samoa

Department of Health
Pago Pago, American Samoa

Department of Health
Pago Pago, American Samoa

South Carolina

South Carolina Commission on Alcohol and Drug Abuse
P.O. Box 4616, Landmark East
3700 Forest Drive
Suite 300
Columbia, South Carolina 29240

South Carolina Commission on Alcohol and Drug Abuse
P.O. Box 4616, Landmark East
3700 Forest Drive
Suite 300
Columbia, South Carolina 29240
Telephone: (803) 758-2521

Officially Designated Authority   *Program Contact*

South Dakota

Department of Health
Foss Building
Pierre, South Dakota 57501

Division of Alcoholism
Office Building No. 2
State Capitol
Pierre, South Dakota 57501
Telephone: (605) 224-3459

Tennessee

Department of Mental Health
300 Cordell Hull Building
Nashville, Tennessee 37219

Section on Alcohol and Drugs
300 Cordell Hull Building
Nashville, Tennessee 37219
Telephone: (615) 741-1921

Texas

Texas Commission on Alcoholism
809 Sam Houston State Office Building
Austin, Texas 78701

Texas Commission on Alcoholism
809 Sam Houston State Office Building
Austin, Texas 78701
Telephone: (512) 475-2577

Trust Territory of the Pacific Islands

Department of Health Services
Office of the High Commissioner
Saipan, Mariana Islands 96950

Division of Mental Health
Saipan, Mariana Islands 96950

Utah

Department of Social Services
State Capitol Building
Room 221
Salt Lake City, Utah 84114

Division of Alcoholism and Drugs
554 South 300 East Street
Salt Lake City, Utah 84114
Telephone: (801) 328-6532

Vermont

Agency of Human Services
Office of the Secretary
State Office Building
Montpelier, Vermont 05602

Alcohol and Drug Abuse Division
81 River Street
Montpelier, Vermont 05602
Telephone: (802) 828-2721

Officially Designated Authority   *Program Contact*

Virgin Islands

Department of Health
Commissioner of Health
P.O. Box 1442
St. Thomas, U.S. Virgin Islands 00801

Mental Health Services
P.O. Box 1442
St. Thomas, U.S. Virgin Islands 00801
Telephone: (809) 774-0117

Virginia

Department of Health
James Madison Building
109 Governor Street
Richmond, Virginia 23219

Bureau of Alcohol Studies and Rehabilitation
James Madison Building
109 Governor Street
Richmond, Virginia 23219
Telephone: (804) 786-3082

Washington

Department of Social and Health Services
Public Lands Building
Olympia, Washington 98504

Office of Alcoholism
Mailstop 45-1
Olympia, Washington 98504
Telephone: (206) 753-5866

West Virginia

Department of Mental Health
State Capitol
Charleston, West Virginia 25305

Division of Alcoholism and Drug Abuse
State Capitol
Charleston, West Virginia 25305
Telephone: (304) 348-3616

Wisconsin

Department of Health and Social Services
1 West Wilson Street
Madison, Wisconsin 53702

Bureau of Alcoholism and Other Drug Abuse
1 West Wilson Street
Madison, Wisconsin 53702
Telephone: (608) 266-3442

Officially Designated Authority   *Program Contact*

Wyoming

Division of Health and Medical Services
State Office Building
Cheyenne, Wyoming 82001

Mental Health and Mental Retardation Services
State Office Building
Cheyenne, Wyoming 82001
Telephone: (307) 777-7351

Appendix VI

Foods to Offer Before Serving Drinks

Cold
French bread with soft cheese (Brie, and so on)
Apple and pear slices with hunks of hard or soft cheese
Thick dips (sour-cream consistency), served with raw carrot sticks, celery, cauliflower flowerets
Plump finger sandwiches with meat, egg, or cheese filling
Deviled eggs

Hot
Blintzes (small pancakes) filled with meat or cheese
Parmesan puffs (equal parts Parmesan cheese and mayonnaise mixed and heated on party rye bread and browned under the broiler)
Meatballs
Cocktail franks wrapped in pastry dough and heated

Avoid
Thirst-producing snack foods (peanuts, potato chips, pretzels)
Vegetables alone
Brittle breads (rye thins, and so on) alone

INDEX

AA, *see* Alcoholics Anonymous
Absinthe, 102
Absorption of alcohol in body, 16
　See also Body
Abstainers, longevity of, 52
Accidents from drinking alcohol, 112
Acenocoumarol, 170
Addiction to alcohol, 35, 37, 64
Addictive personalities, 27
Addresses of alcoholism authorities and contacts, 174-85
Advertisements for alcohol, 88
After-dinner drinks, 156
Age for drinking, legal, 100
Alcohol abuse, definition of, 112
Alcoholic content, 171
Alcoholics
　nature of, 107-8
　number of, 76-77
　See also Recovered alcoholics
Alcoholics Anonymous (AA), 116, 117-19
　drinks at meetings of, 40
Alcoholism, 105-28
　addresses of programs vs., 174-85
　cause of, 109-10
　cure for, 24-25, 116-17, 123
　definition of, 76, 112
　as illness, 105-6, 119
　nature of, 105
　prevention of, 126-28
　recovery from, 116; *see also* Recovered alcoholics
　treatment for, 117-23
　whether treatment is needed for, 121-22
　See also specific topics
Aldomet, 166
American Indians, alcoholism among, 77-78
American Medical Association, 53
American value system, drinking and, 74

Amount of alcohol
　to cause tipsiness, 45-46
　metabolized per hour, 28, 37
　safe, 16-17, 32-33
　used by average American, 74-75
　of various drinks, compared, 35-36
Amount of money spent on alcohol, 75-76
Amphetamine, 168, 170
Analgesic drugs, 169
Analgesic properties of alcohol, 53
Anesthetic, alcohol as, 16, 32, 48, 54, 104, 173
Anesthetic drugs, 169
Angina pectoris, 53
Anstie's Law, 16-17
　alcohol abuse as drinking more than, 112
Antabuse, 122, 166, 169
Antibiotics, 165
Anticoagulant drugs, 170
Anticonvulsant drugs, 170
Antidepressants, 167, 170
Antidiabetic drugs, 169
Antifreeze, 36
Antihistamines, 64, 165-66, 196
Antihypertensive drugs, 166, 170
Anxiety, 127
　in heart patient, alcohol and, 53
Aperitifs, 171
Aphrodisiac
　absinthe as, 102
　alchohol as, 22
Appetite, alcohol as stimulator of, 33, 41, 54, 68
Apresoline, 166
Aspirin, 49
　alcohol and, 64-65, 169
Arentyl, 167

Barbiturates, 64, 168, 170
Bars, 156-57, 159

Beer, 34, 36
  alcohol content of, 171
  alcohol content, compared, 35
  amount drunk by average American, 75
  amount to serve, 156
  glasses for, 154
  with whiskey, 29
Beer belly, cause of, 42
Beer parties, college, 91
Benadryl, 169
Benefits of alcohol, 11-14
Bible, the, wine in, 68
Blackouts, 113
Bladder, full, 43, 44
Blood alcohol concentrations, effect of, 172-73
Bloodstream, alcohol's entry into, 16, 17, 34, 36
Blue Cross, 119
Body
  how alcohol works in, 16, 17
  how fast alcohol works in, 34
Body weight
  alcohol's effect and, 32-33
  diet for loss of, and alcohol, 41
  gain in, and alcohol, 40
Boilermaker, 29
Booths, heavier drinking in, 156
Bottle, marking of, 159
Brain
  alcohol and damage to, 37
  alcohol's effect on, 16, 32, 34, 38, 60
Brain cells, killing of, supposedly by alcohol, 28
Brandy, 34, 156
Bromides, 170
Business
  alcohol in, 82, 85
  losses of, caused by alcoholism, 86
  and prevention of alcoholism, 127-28

Caffeine, 28, 168, 170
Calcium carbamide, 169
Calories, alcoholic
  compared to food, 33
  of ounce of absolute alcohol, 40
Canada, 101
Cancer, alcohol and, 37
Carbonated mixers, 34, 50, 155
Central nervous system depressants
  alcohol as, 32
  other drugs as, 165, 167, 168
Children, 88-91
  of alcoholic parents, 89-90
  drinking by, 88-89

  explanations to, 160-61
China, 18
Chinese in U.S., 78-79
Chloral hydrates, 168
Chloromycetin, 165
Churchill, Winston, 11, 13, 14
Cirrhosis of the liver, 57
Closeness to other people, alcohol and, 61
Cocktail lounges, 156-57
Cocktail parties, 18, 70
Codeine, 169
Coffee, for sobering up, 28
Cold shower, for sobering up, 28
College students, beer parties by, 91
Coma, alcoholic, 32, 173
Companions
  for drinking, 19, 68-69
  heavy drinkers as, 26
Compazine, 167
Congeners, hangovers and, 50
Congress, alcoholism and, 84
Contac, 169
Control, and effect of drinking, 44-45, 46, 61
Cordials, alcohol content of, 171
Coricidin, 169
Cost of alcoholism in U.S., 86
Cost of drinking, 101
Crime, alcohol and, 37
Cure for alcoholism, 116-17, 123
  whether there is a, 24-25

Darvon, 165
Demerol, 165, 169
Denatured alcohol, 36
Denmark, 122
Dependence on alcohol, 61
Depressants, *see* Central nervous system depressants
Depression, when increased by drinking, 60
Deserpidine, 170
Diabinese, 166
Diaries, drinking, 130-52
Diazepam, 170
Digestion, alcohol as aid to, 54
Dilantin, 165, 170
Dialudid, 165
"Diluted," in federal law, 36
Dilution of drinks, 34, 154
Disease, alcohol and, 37, 52
Distilled spirits
  alcohol content of, 171
  amount drunk by average American, 75
  amount to serve, 155-56

188 / INDEX

Disulfiram (Antabuse), 122, 166
Diuretic drugs, 166, 170
Doctors, *see* Physicians
Doxepin, 170
Dralzine, 166
Drinking problem
  definitions of, 112
  of drinker who insists he doesn't have problem, 121
  friends with, 161, 163
  getting drink as sign of, 113
  helping spouse with, 161-62
  need of help for, 132
  signs of, 112-13
  social drinking distinguished from, 12
Drinking records, personal (drinking diaries), 130-52
Driving and drinking, 96-97
Drugs and alcohol together, 64-65, 165-70
Drunkenness (tipsiness)
  amount of alcohol needed for, 45-46
  coating stomach with milk to prevent, 27
  of companion, what to do, 163
  condonation of, 108-9
  degrees of, 172-73
  every time one drinks, 113
  at parties, 70
  spree of, as danger to health, 56
  symptoms of, 32
"Dry mouth," alcohol and, 54

Education about alcohol, 88
Elavil, 167
Elderly, the, alcohol and, 53
Employees, handling drinking by, 162-63
Epilepsy, use of Dilantin for, and alcohol, 165
Esimil, 166
Ethyl alcohol, 36
Eytony, 167

Families, alcoholism in, 22-23
Famous people
  alcoholism and, 83-84
  spouses of, 84
Fat, floating, in the blood, 55-56
Federal law on alcoholic content, 35-36
Fields, W. C., 43
First drink, alcoholics from, 106-7
Food
  alcohol and, 17, 34-35
  appetite for, and alcohol, 33, 41, 54, 68
  calories of, compared to alcohol calories, 33
  enhanced by alcohol, 68
  at parties, 69, 186
  types of, to serve with drinking, 154
France, 74, 75, 78
Friends with drinking problems, 161, 163
Friendship, drinking and, 69

Glasses, types of, to use, 154
Group drinking, 69
Guanethidine, 170
Guests, drinks for, 154-58

Handling people who want you to drink, 162
Hangovers, 48-50
  avoidance of, 49, 50
  definition of, 48
  drinks for purpose of killing, 26-27
  reason for, 48-49
  switching drinks and, 50
  treatment of, 49, 50
Hay-fever medication, 169
Heart disease, alcohol and, 52-53
Heavy drinkers
  adverse physical effects of, 56-57
  association with, 26
  "alcoholics" compared to, 109
  definition of, 113
  nutrition and, 56
  who do not get tipsy, 46
Hemingway, Ernest, 102
Heredity, alcoholism and, 22-23
Heroin, 35, 100-1
"High," meaning of, 37-38
Hosting, 155-56
Housewives, drinking problems of, 84
How to drink, 17
Hunger suppressant, alcohol as, 33-34
Hypoglycemia, 166
Hypotension, 45

Ice cubes, use of, 155
Imipramine, 170
India, prohibition in, 127
Information about alcoholism, 104
Insulin, oral, 166-69
Intelligence, alcohol and, 28
Irish, alcoholism among, 77-78
Ismelin, 166
Isopropyl alcohol, 37
Italians in U.S., 78-79
Italy, 75, 78

Japan, 77
Jews, 78-79

Khrushchev, Nikita, 101
Koran, the, 127

Legal restrictions on drinking, 100-1
Liquor industry, sales aim of, 88
Liver
  cirrhosis of, 57
  drinking and, 55
Loneliness, alcohol and, 19, 40, 127
Longevity of drinkers, 52
Lunch, drinks at, 16, 82

Marijuana, alcohol compared to, 37, 90
Marplan, 167
Mecalymine, 170
Medication
  alcohol as, 53
  effects of, when combined with alcohol, 165-70
Mellaril, 167
Meperidine, 169
Meprobamate, 170
Methadone, 169
"Mickey Finn," 168
Military services, drinking problems in, 82-83
Minors, drinking by, 100
Mixed drinks, 154, 155
  carbonation and, 34, 50, 155
Moderate drinking
  health and, 52-53
  sex and, 41-42
  upper limit of, 16, 126
Money, amount of, spent on alcohol, 75-76
Monoamine-oxidase inhibitors, 170
Morphine, 169
Music, type of, when drinking, 155

Narcotic drugs, 169
Nardil, 167
Nation, Carry, 13
National Council on Alcoholism, 117
National Institute on Alcohol Abuse and Alcoholism, 11
Need for alcohol, 112, 113
"Needing" a drink, 61
Norpramin, 167
Number of alcoholics, 76-77, 109
Number of persons who drink, 76
Nutrition, *see* Food

Occasional drinkers, 76
Offering a drink, ways of, 157
Oral stimulation, 40
Orinase, 166

Overdrinking, prevention of, 158-59
Oxygen for hangovers, 49

Paraphernalia for drinking, 154
Parties
  cocktail, 18, 70
  differences in drinking at, 69-70
  discussions after, 160
  foods at, 69, 186
  rules for, 154-58
  substitutes for drinks at, 158
Peer pressure for drinking, 70-71
Pharmacologic action of alcohol, 32
Phenidamine, 170
Phenothiazines, 167, 170
Physicians
  alcoholism among, 83
  treatment of alcoholism by, 120-21
Pictures of drinkers, 159
Pneumonia, 53
Poe, Edgar Allan, 83
Polydipsia, 40
Pot, *see* Marijuana
Potato chips, 154
Powerful people, alcoholism and, 83-84
Premature ejaculation, 22
Preparation of drinks, 154, 157
Pretzels, 154
Problem drinking, *see* Drinking problem
Problem-solving, alcohol and, 28
Professions, alcohol and, 85
Prohibition, failure of, 127
Prolixin, 167

Quinthazone, 170

Recovered alcoholics
  drinking again by, 25, 108
  drinking in presence of, 107
  whether still alcoholic, 107
Red nose, cause of, 42-43
Refusing drinks, 159, 161
Regular drinkers, number of, 76
Religion, alcohol and, 68, 71
Relaxation
  as purpose of drinking, 60
  when drinking, 155
REM sleep, alcohol and, 55
Repoise, 167
Reserpine, 166, 170
Responsible drinking, 19-20
Rubbing alcohol, 37

Safe amount of alcohol, 16-17, 32-33
Salicylates, 64-65. 169

Salty snacks, 154
Sedatives, alcohol and, 64, 168, 170
Sex, alcohol and, 22, 40, 41-42, 69
Shyness, drinking and, 68
Sinequan, 167
Sleep, alcohol to induce, 55
Sobering up, whether there is a quick way for, 28
Social drinking, problem drinking distinguished from, 12
Social upheaval, increasing of drinking during, 60
Soviet Union, 74, 91, 101
Spirits, *see* Distilled spirits
Spouses with drinking problems, 84, 161-62
Spree drinkers, 113
State borders and drinking by minors, 100
Stomach
   absorption of alcohol by, 16, 34
   coating of, with milk, to prevent drunkenness, 27
   irritation of, with alcohol, 34, 54
   salicylates and, 64-65
Substitutes for drinks, 158
Sulfanamids, 165
Sweden, 74, 91
Sweets, gorging on, after stopping drinking, 44

Tape recordings of drinkers, 159
Teenagers, 90, 91
Television, 85, 88, 128
Tension, overdrinking from, 156
Tension-producing work, alcoholism and, 85
Thiazide, 170
Thirst
   drinking and, 43
   from pretzels, etc., 154
Thorazine, 167
Thujone, 102
Tight deadlines, alcoholism and, 85
Tindal, 167
Tipsiness, *see* Drunkenness
Tofränil, 167
Tranquilizers, 167, 168, 170
Treatment for alcoholism, 117-23
Tuberculosis, 109-10

Ulcers, drinking with, 54
"Uptight" drinking, 44, 46, 49

Valium, 168
Vasodilation, 42, 45
Vermouth, 102, 171
Vitamins, alcohol and, 170
Vodka, alcoholic content of, 35

Washington (D.C.), use of alcohol in, 74-75
Water
   as mixer, 155
   as unsafe, 74, 78
Weight, *see* Body weight
When to drink, 17-18
Where to drink, 18
"Whirlies," 45
Whiskey, 36
   with beer, 29
   See also Distilled spirits
Wilde, Oscar, 41
Wine, 34
   to aid digestion, 54
   alcoholic content of, 35, 191
   amount drunk by average American, 75
   amount to serve, 156
   enhancement of food by, 68
   in France, 74
   glasses for, 154
   red vs. white, in making you sick, 28-29
Women
   alcoholism of, 22-23, 84
   safe amount of alcohol for, 33
Wormwood, 102
Writers, alcoholics among, 83

Young people, use of alcohol by, 90-91
   in other countries, 91